T0143343

Medical History Education for Health Practitioners

LISETTA LOVETT
BSc, DHMSA, FRCPsych
Honorary Senior Lecturer
School of Humanities, Keele University

and

ALANNAH TOMKINS
DPhil, FRHS
Senior Lecturer in History
School of Humanities, Keele University

Foreword by
PAUL LAZARUS
President
Association for Medical Humanities

Illustrations by
MOULI XIONG AND JOANNE PRESCOTT

Radcliffe Publishing
London • New York

Radcliffe Publishing Ltd
33–41 Dallington Street
London
EC1V 0BB
United Kingdom

www.radcliffehealth.com

© 2013 Lisetta Lovett and Alannah Tomkins

Lisetta Lovett and Alannah Tomkins have asserted their right under the Copyright, Designs and Patents Act 1988 to be identified as the authors of this work.

Every effort has been made to ensure that the information in this book is accurate. This does not diminish the requirement to exercise clinical judgement, and neither the publisher nor the authors can accept any responsibility for its use in practice.

All rights reserved. No part of this publication may be reproduced, stored in a retrieval system or transmitted, in any form or by any means, electronic, mechanical, photocopying, recording or otherwise, without the prior permission of the copyright owner.

British Library Cataloguing in Publication Data

A catalogue record for this book is available from the British Library.

ISBN-13: 978 184619 981 3

Typeset by Darkriver Design, Auckland, New Zealand
Printed and bound by Cadmus Communications, USA

Contents

Contents

Foreword

IMAGINE WE ARE SETTING OUT ON A LONG AND TORTUOUS JOURNEY by road to a destination that we have never been to before. On the way, we find ourselves at a complex junction and realise we are lost. How do we decide which route to follow? We can, of course, use our knowledge of where our destination might lie and our skills in reading maps and/or operating our in-car navigation system. However, we might be able to make a more informed decision about which road to choose if we could understand how we managed to arrive at our current location in the first place.

Twenty-first century medicine is just the current stage of a never-ending journey of tremendous complexity. Those of us who are fortunate enough to practise in this day and age do so in ways that are themselves the results of huge changes over many centuries – advances in areas such as medication and surgical and imaging techniques and developments in our understanding of the human body and its attendant threats through genetics. Add to that list the huge social and societal changes in public health, attitudes to illness and changes in ethical viewpoints, and we find ourselves at the current forefront of medical evolution but nowhere near the end of this particular journey. We also find ourselves struggling to make meaning of many of these changes and how to deploy them with the best interests of our patients at heart. Maybe the knowledge, skills and attitudes that our teachers urged us to develop and that we continue to nurture throughout our professional lives are by themselves not enough. We need to understand how and why we have got to this particular point in the history of medicine in the first place to make the best decisions and to tolerate the ambiguities and uncertainties that clinical practice throws at us daily.

Let us now return to our road journey. We have resolved our navigational dilemma, and have stopped to admire the surrounding countryside. We look around in awe, taking in the sights around us. However, this feeling of wonderment may be magnified by our recollection of the journey we have undertaken so far – by the towns, river valleys, hills and mountains that we passed through and over to get here. Today's medical practitioners often pause with similar thoughts about what has gone before us as well as the changes that have taken place during our own time. This produces our own professional wonderment – something that makes us appreciate even more what we have now and spurs us on to make full use of this knowledge and extend the boundaries of practice even further. The history of our craft, of how we got to where we are today – the inheritances from our professional forebears that still work for us and the discredited theories and abandoned practices of past times – make the myriad of facts that we have to know for present-day practice more understandable. For many, learning this makes practice that much more enjoyable as well. Encouraging parallel, divergent, reflective thoughts and processes alongside the rational, scientific rules that we need to follow fosters a deeper understanding of what we learn under the banner of medicine and how comfortably or uncomfortably this knowledge now sits in the delivery of everyday clinical practice. Thus, we would do well to remember that medicine itself is a journey and knowing something of its history helps us travel along it by giving a fuller meaning to our current position, whether we have stopped because we are lost or merely to admire the scenery.

Paul Lazarus
President, Association for Medical Humanities
Centre for Medical Humanities, University of Leicester
June 2013

About the authors

Lisetta Lovett is a retired National Health Service consultant psychiatrist and senior lecturer in medical education. She undertook a diploma in the history of medicine while a medical student at Guy's Hospital. She has published on the 'madhouse keeper' Thomas Bakewell and two online modules on the history of mental health legislation for the Royal College of Psychiatrists. She has written a chapter for a book about the neuronovel, *Syndrome Syndrome*, and co-authored a book on medical ethics. She introduced medical humanities to Keele University's School of Medicine and made provision for a wide range of titles for student-selected components. She continues to co-organise a master's module on medical humanities for qualified doctors. She is now an honorary senior lecturer in the School of Humanities at Keele.

Alannah Tomkins is a senior lecturer in history at Keele University. She has been researching and teaching the history of medicine for the last 20 years and has published on infirmaries, man-midwives and mad doctors. She has taught on the Keele Bachelor of Medicine, Bachelor of Surgery programme since 2003 and offers medical humanities student-selected components to undergraduates. She is currently writing a book, which is provisionally titled 'Disappointed Doctors: medical career turbulence in an age of professionalisation, 1780–1890'.

Acknowledgements

MANY PEOPLE HAVE ASSISTED WITH THE PROVISION OF HISTORICAL material and examples for this book, not least our colleagues and the students who have studied the history of medicine with us over the last decade. In particular, we would like to credit and thank James Blackburn, Jennie Hubbard, Alistair Moulden, Harriet May Parker, Kim Price and Melissa White.

For Jonathan, patient and long-suffering husband, best friend and
critic, who sustained me with his support and encouragement.
Also for my sons Tomos, for suggesting that I buy a Mac, and
Adam, for his critical comments about my writing style.

LL

For Lola, who hasn't had a book yet.

AT

Abbreviations

AHA	area health authority
DHA	district health authority
GP	general practitioner
HIV	human immunodeficiency virus
MMR	measles, mumps and rubella
NHS	National Health Service
NICE	National Institute for Health and Care Excellence
NSPCC	National Society for the Prevention of Cruelty to Children
PTSD	post-traumatic stress disorder
RHA	regional health authority
RoSPA	Royal Society for the Prevention of Accidents
UK	United Kingdom
USA	United States of America
WHO	World Health Organization

Introduction

Medical history and the medical humanities: the definition of a discipline

This book has arisen from a keen desire to establish an amiable and respectful dialogue between groups that form uneasy alliances in academia or easily drift apart. This should be an uncontroversial (if complex) agenda. Unfortunately it is not.

In September 2012, Imperial College London decided to close its Centre for the History of Science, Technology and Medicine. The centre was ranked as the top history department for research in the United Kingdom (UK) in 2008, but this was not enough to secure its future at Imperial College. Instead, the college transferred its former staff to King's College London, citing concerns about the centre's small size and the challenges it would face in maintaining its standing. One professor at Imperial College was more specific, and notably criticised the centre's staff for being too insular, so depriving them of a higher profile within their home institution. In other words, the history researchers had excelled to national and international acclaim but had neglected the nonetheless marginal tenure they enjoyed at a predominantly scientific university.

This is one example among many possible instances of how different disciplines fail to communicate with one another, to the detriment of one or both sides. CP Snow's 'two cultures' are possibly as oppositional as they ever were.[1] Dialogue between medicine and history will take place, just as the broader debate between the arts and sciences will continue, if only because no discipline exists alone. However, the weight given to each side will depend heavily on context, and researchers trained in one discipline rather than both will tend to give a natural preference to the methods and discipline most familiar to them. At the same time, there is abundant evidence that uncertainty about an alien discipline encourages people to be either over-confident and flippant or suspicious and derogatory about methods that they do not understand or for which they cannot determine the value. The tenor of the dialogue is frequently tetchy, defensive or resentful.

This becomes particularly obvious when an expert in one discipline has the courage or temerity to attempt competence in another. If a medical practitioner turns their hand to history, they are not always welcomed or become perplexed by the demands of historical prose. If an academic historian ventures to offer insights on runs of medical statistics, they risk being misinterpreted or quickly dismissed.

It is almost unheard of for a professional historian to change career and become an employed doctor, but, if they did, they would inherently acquire a new set of research approaches. Neil Vickers, co-founder of the first British master of arts course in literature and medicine at King's College London, has academic qualifications in literature but became a research fellow in epidemiology at St George's Hospital Medical School in 1991.[2] Tentative steps in any direction are an easy target for charges of lack of information, stifling detail, inadequate analysis or unrefined conclusions.[3]

Successful crossover is possible but is more evident via individual doctors' immersion in history and in the United States of America (USA) rather than Britain. Twentieth-century surveys of American medical education 'lamented the minimalist presence of history', while the expansion of specifically medical history in the second half of the century tended to distance it from medical students.[3] The result is a very patchy acknowledgement of the potential for history to affect practice. Jacalyn Duffin's book *Clio in the Clinic: history in medical practice*[4] offers 23 essays by practitioner-historians united, in the view of Chris Feudtner, by their intimate tone and their practical application of historical insight in a clinical context. Nonetheless, the overall impression is idiosyncratic and kaleidoscopic rather than comprehensive or coherent.[5] The future for history in American medicine is more secure, in that nearly half of medical schools' curricula included humanities options in 2002.[6]

In Britain, the publication of *Tomorrow's Doctors: recommendations on undergraduate medical education* in 1993 gave an obvious steer to medical schools by emphasising the presence of humanities optional modules to improve communication skills and reflectivity.[7] Recent editions of 2003 and 2009 have somewhat retreated from this early commitment, but perhaps this is because student-selected components have become so widely adopted in British medical curricula.

Medical history as a component of medical humanities

Medical history holds an important place in the composite medical humanities. The portmanteau nature of 'humanities' means that it can legitimately be used to refer to highly diverse and simultaneously specialised activities. It can cover esoteric ethical inquiry that is purely philosophical, or practical arts interventions for patient groups, and a multitude of variants on the non-scientific disciplines and the practice of creative arts. Anything that pertains to 'humanity' rather than to the biomedical sciences may be incorporated. The Association of Medical Humanities was launched in Britain in 2002, and medical humanities came of age in Britain in 2008 with the establishment of two academic centres – one at King's College London and the other at Durham University – with nearly £4 million of funding from the Wellcome Trust.

However, history is special, first because it is 'the oldest humanities subject involved with medical education' and second because sincere claims can be made for the magnitude of its impact.[3] Without a shadow of irony, Felipe Fernández-Armesto has summarised the potential of the discipline of history thus:

There are only two good reasons to study anything: to enhance life and prepare for death. History enhances life by giving us the thrill of making sense of experience: seeing more vividly the landscapes and streetscapes that surround us, perceiving more deeply the people we meet, glimpsing the images and hearing the sounds we encounter more richly because we know the past they come from. It prepares us for death by giving us some basic moral equipment: the ability, or at least the willingness, to shift our perspective and defer to what historians call 'the sources' – the representations of themselves others have left for us. If you can make the effort to understand people in remoter periods of your own culture, let alone those of others, you will be more likely to sympathise with alterity in your own times ...[8]

Since doctors and patients are usually divided by power and knowledge (as well as sometimes by class and culture), the value of historical study in medical contexts is, we hope, tangible. The remainder of this introduction describes some of these benefits in more detail.

Why is this relevant to health professionals?

Popular journalism would hold that study of humanities disciplines is designed to make health professionals more, well, humane.[9] This entails diverting the professional gaze away from the technologies of biomedical science towards the social/cultural contexts of the disease/injury experience. However, compassion, empathy and humanity cannot be taught and their uptake cannot be tested. The reality is much more complicated but also much more rewarding than easy generalities imply.

There is a school of thought that suggests medical history is most useful when confined to the recent past and to the circumstances of technological change. In this vein, the utility of history to the clinician would be to tell her or him about what happened *last*, and what their predecessors did, before the most recent modes of practice were forged.[10] While this stance offers a quick and obvious way for history to appear relevant to medical education and policy, it is unnecessarily reductive. It implies that historical understanding is only relevant when it is informing immediate pressures on institutions, welfare systems or governments, and elides the fact that medicine is not synonymous with health, just as doctors cannot be said to speak for patients. Even a cursory consideration of the field reveals that a longer view is required. Medicine is essentially a reactive science, in that it responds to patients' presentments. In the twenty-first century world, this entails addressing many degenerative diseases, while, in earlier times, practitioners were faced instead with fast-acting infectious diseases. The media is always keen to remind the first-world public that this emphasis may return in the event of a new pandemic (possibly of an influenza virus strain). In this event, historical epidemiology and palaeopathology may be key to an understanding of how, for example, leprosy changed from being a 'slow-moving Old World disease' to a 'global scourge within a few hundred years'.[11]

Habits of reflection are patently encouraged in all of the medical professions, and reflective writing is embedded in formal summative assessment in some courses. This may appear to encourage mechanical compliance among beginning students, but, ideally, recruits will learn to see the value of honest self-reflection as a tool to support (rather than undermine) their professional identity. Reflective learning, followed by reflective practice, may aspire to offer career-long avenues for refreshment and aid practitioners in avoiding of unhelpful and entrenched attitudes and practices.

Study of medical history can assist the practitioner to become more sensitive to the social context in which human values are formed and understand behaviours that might otherwise appear antisocial or inexplicable. In her highly successful best-selling book *Call the Midwife: a true story of the East End in the 1950s*, Jennifer Worth (1935–2011) reflected on her experiences with a patient known as 'Lil'. The patient in this instance presented with a demeanour that Worth found extremely off-putting, given that she was clearly amused by her visit to maternity services and quite casual in accepting the news that she had venereal disease 'again'. This patient encounter meant that Worth was apprehensive of making a home visit but on seeing the squalor of the tenements that Lil called home, she became much less judgemental.[12] What we do not know, of course, is how long it took Worth to arrive at a more moderate assessment of her patient, given that her memoirs were written after retirement.

At its most basic, this sort of sensitivity can assist practitioners to cross the divide and become active advocates for the patient perspective. At its most radical, study of medical history and other humanities may inspire a wholly liberated intellectual response against the 'tyranny of expertise'.[13]

Acceptance of ambiguity is a particularly difficult adjustment for people with a predominantly scientific disciplinary background. This is ironic and paradoxical in medicine, given the notional authority of the generic practitioners *versus* the uncertainties inevitable in specific cases. History provides illustrations of medical 'failures' which, rather than undermining practitioners in the present day, can encourage a healthy, sceptical and informed perspective on the changing understandings of medical 'knowledge'.[3] The need for such a lack of certainty has been revealed relatively recently. Ian Kennedy's 1981 book *The Unmasking of Medicine* endeavours to show that definitions of 'disease', 'illness' and 'health' are not static or morally neutral.[14] This seems a relatively uncontentious idea now, but was met with vituperation in the early 1980s, much of which emanated from the medical profession. Yet the condition of not always having an answer to a problem or question is an entirely normal part of human life.[15]

An awareness of historical time can foster and enhance a tentative or provisional acceptance of scientific knowledge. This stance is well suited to twenty-first century medicine, in which change is rapid and techniques and technologies might be outmoded swiftly. This is not to say that we should endorse an ultra-critical response to all new research and clinical findings. David Wootton's book *Bad Medicine: doctors doing harm since Hippocrates* takes doctors to task for their 'failure' to devise and promote antisepsis sooner, but this is both unnecessarily demoralising and anachronistic.[16] People of the past cannot reasonably be chastised for failing to be more 'modern', if only because a historical perspective will encourage a measure of self-protection among most thinking people. What criticisms will be made hereafter of the early twenty-first century? There is no need to feel crushed by the knowledge that we do not yet know what we do not know – but it is sensible to admit that there are still plenty of medical revelations, realisations and developments to come.

Finally, if the value of medical history is not solely pragmatic, neither is it entirely esoteric. History provides concrete examples for action and decision in a present-centred policy context. At the time of writing, access to innovative treatments is limited in Britain by the National Institute for Health and Care Excellence (NICE). Many of its decisions are not at all beneficial for patients – for example, when the institute deems a treatment too costly to be extended as an option to all potentially-eligible patients. Most people would freely and democratically subscribe to the idea that healthcare spending cannot be limitless; there must be some regulatory framework to weigh treatment benefits with hard financial costs. Decisions are made by NICE alone; if challenged, then resolution is sought in the courts; wholesale opposition would require parliamentary inquiry. However, to address questions of entitlement, NICE employees, judges, justices and parliamentarians can only turn to humanities subjects like history. This does not mean that the contribution of academics is acknowledged or rewarded, in Britain or elsewhere. In the Supreme Court of the United States, '[o]ne landmark case contained a long paragraph about religious liberties that defined American constitutional law for decades. It had been lifted, nearly verbatim and without attribution, from a history professor's book'.[17] In other words, while scientific medicine may provide us with the technical means to address the most stubborn diseases, it may still pose new questions, to which only history may hold the answers.

The skills of the student trained in humanities subjects cannot be feigned; regrettably, though, the value of medical history to training and practising professionals is not always championed, and if clinicians do not value the disciplines that collectively address the psychosocial aspects of medicine, students will quickly adopt similar views. As some American students have bluntly expressed, they 'don't see clinicians referencing that stuff' and 'just don't have time for that now. There is no pay-off'.[18] It is unlikely that any conceivable sequence of events would, overnight, encourage practitioners or trainees to become attentive to medical humanities. We hope that this book helps to make incremental progress in the task of reframing the significance of humanities, generally, and history, specifically, for medical professionals.

Whose medical history?

This book deals chiefly with the history of medicine in Britain since 1600. When relevant, it refers to medical historical practice and insights before 1600 and in different cultures. Medical advances are often attributed to great men but were possibly more the result of prevailing social, economic and cultural factors that facilitated prepared minds to be innovative. To help contextualise these advances, this book will inform the reader of some of those factors.

Many of the readers of this book will work for the British National Health Service (NHS) at some point in their careers, if not for the entirety of their working life. The NHS dates from 5 July 1948, when the majority of existing hospitals (built under the auspices of either the English Poor Laws or the efforts of individual charities) entered public ownership. The institution is regarded as a national triumph and an occasion for unified, mutual congratulation. The intermittent focus on the NHS in the opening ceremony of the London Olympic Games in July 2012 was widely approved in Britain (if not always appreciated elsewhere).

Its origins were much less consensual. The lay and medical political establishments were fiercely opposed to the NHS initially, and it has remained a central feature of party-political dispute ever since. To understand the NHS and to participate in future changes, clinicians, who are frequently exhorted to be more involved in NHS management, are likely to benefit from having a historical awareness of its antecedents, genesis and evolution to the present day. We have included some chapters that explicitly trace the professionalisation of some health disciplines and the history of the NHS and its managers, but we also hope that the book's content is more generally informative on the history of medicine in Britain for sometime or full-time employees of the NHS.

How to use this book

Although this book is intended for health tutors, students and qualified health practitioners may use it for their own interest. There are two ways this book can be used by tutors. For the most part, they may wish to use it as a quick source of information in their subject area – be it cardiovascular disease, emergency medicine or child protection – to provide historical context, interest and sometimes entertainment for their tutees. Alternatively, they may wish to use the book as the basis of a programme of seminars on the history of medicine. With the latter possibility in mind, we need to stress that this book does not attempt to be a comprehensive text on the entire history of medicine. Further, it is biased towards the history of Western medicine after 1600, although there are certainly references to other cultures and epochs to provide a more balanced overview and encourage the interested student to read more. One of the book's main aims is simply to provide some historical background to health topics that students in most health disciplines will encounter in their core training as well as to foster in them a further appreciation of wider health issues. The topics covered were originally suggested to us by a medical undergraduate problem-based learning curriculum that is employed in a number of medical schools for the first 2 years of study. We have subsequently expanded into other areas chosen to provide supplementary historical information to other chapters. Consequently, the first five sections address mostly mainstream clinical issues. Section 1, 'Emergency!', addresses health at crisis points. 'The pleasures of life' examines the historical background to diet and dieting, misuse of drugs and alcohol, and sex. The next section, 'The facts of life' provides an overview of women's issues, health and medicine, while Section 4, 'Infection, immunity and public health', concentrates on tuberculosis and influenza, explaining why it took so long to reach an understanding of how infection is spread and to discover methods of control such as vaccination. Public health is also about social attitudes and economic forces, so we have included the subject of child labour and welfare in this section. The next section, 'The challenges of life', covers disability, mental illness, child safeguarding and finally ageing and death. The next two sections are devoted to the practise of medicine. The first chapter of Section 6 describes medicine in the ancient Graeco-Roman era as well as the development of humoral theory and how this became so influential. The remaining chapters in this section concentrate on the evolution of modern diagnosis by describing some of the developments that helped practitioners to break out of the stranglehold of Galenic doctrine. Section 7 is about the history of a range of medical interventions, some highly successful and some destined to be recognised as misdirection. The final section, 'Healers and health carers', addresses the history of health services pre and post the NHS and the professionalisation of some of our health disciplines.

The chapters within each section have been kept short so they can be quickly assimilated. They can be dipped into, since each is self-contained, but there are cross-references to other chapters that the interested reader may wish to pursue. Most chapters have suggested questions to pose to students that may assist group discussion; putative answers are available at the end of the book. Although this book primarily offers a historical account, there are references on occasion to literature, art and medicine that a tutor may wish to use to widen discussion. To facilitate further reflection and discussion, each chapter ends with some comments about why having a grasp of the historical context of that topic is relevant today and/or of interest.

For students or practitioners of a health discipline, we hope this book will stimulate an interest in history of medicine and lead to further reading. At the very least, the reader may find that the ability to offer a historical perspective in conversation, be it while waiting for results on a ward, scrubbing up in theatre or at a job interview, may enhance his or her interest to colleagues; not all health practitioners want to talk about health all the time! Ideally, we hope that having some historical awareness will allow readers to have a new perspective on their health organisation, other disciplines and the patients with whom he or she works.

Finally, a point in our own defence: we are fully aware that some readers will be surprised that we have not written about certain health topics. To have aimed for comprehensiveness would have defeated the object of this book. However, if there proves to be an adequate number of sorely missed omissions we may be encouraged to consider a sequel!

References

1. Snow CP. *The Two Cultures and the Scientific Revolution*. New York: Cambridge University Press; 1960.
2. Sebba A. A novel take on healing the sick. *Times Higher Education*. 18 March 2005: 18. Available at: www.timeshighereducation.co.uk/features/a-novel-take-on-healing-the-sick/194837.article (accessed 19 April 2013).
3. Dolan B. History, medical humanities and medical education. *Social History of Medicine*. 2010; **23**(2): 393–405.
4. Duffin J, editor. *Clio in the Clinic: history in medical practice*. Oxford: Oxford University Press; 2005.
5. Feudtner JC. Clio in the Clinic: history in medical practice (review). *Bulletin of the History of Medicine*. 2007; **81**(2): 495–6.
6. Strickland MA, Gambala CT, Rodenhauser P. Medical education and the arts: a survey of US medical schools. *Teaching and Learning in Medicine*. 2002; **14**(4): 264–7.
7. General Medical Council. *Tomorrow's Doctors: recommendations on undergraduate medical education*. London: General Medical Council; 1993. Available at: www.gmc-uk.org/Tomorrows_Doctors_1993.pdf_25397206.pdf (accessed 19 April 2013).
8. Fernández-Armesto F. 1588 and all that. *Times Higher Education*. 9 June 2009: 27. Available at: www.timeshighereducation.co.uk/comment/columnists/1588-and-all-that/406945.article (accessed 19 April 2013).
9. NHS docs study art to become more humane. *Times Higher Education*. 5 November 1999: 2. Available at: www.timeshighereducation.co.uk/news/nhs-docs-study-art-to-become-more-humane/148673.article (accessed 19 April 2013).
10. Peckham R. The history of medicine: challenges and futures. *Perspectives on History*. November 2010. Available at: www.historians.org/perspectives/issues/2010/1011/1011fie1.cfm (accessed 19 April 2013).
11. Green M. 'History of medicine' or 'History of health'? *Past and Future*. 2011; **9**(Spring/Summer): 7–9.
12. Worth J. *Call the Midwife: a true story of the East End in the 1950s*. Twickenham: Merton Books; 2002.
13. Pellegrino E. Viewpoints in the teaching of medical history. VII. Medical history and medical education: points of engagement. *Clio Medica*. 1975; **10**(4): 295–303.
14. Kennedy I. *The Unmasking of Medicine*. London: Allen and Unwin; 1981.
15. van Deemter K. *Not Exactly: in praise of vagueness*. Oxford: Oxford University Press; 2010.
16. Wootton D. *Bad Medicine: doctors doing harm since Hippocrates*. Oxford: Oxford University Press; 2007.
17. Drakeman DL. Solid grounding: the humanities roots that support our STEMs. *Times Higher Education*. 20 May 2010: 31. Available at: www.timeshighereducation.co.uk/news/solid-grounding-the-humanities-roots-that-support-our-stems/411655.article (accessed 19 April 2013).
18. Lindberg M, Greene G. Why do they ignore it? Getting students in a PBL curriculum to pay attention to important learning issues that do not appear to them to be central. In: Schwartz P, Menin S, Webb G, editors. *Problem-Based Learning: case studies, experience and practice*. London: Routledge; 2001. pp. 83–9.

Section 1

Emergency!

1

Heroic patients

'HEROIC SURGERY' IS A TERM TRADITIONALLY APPLIED TO AGGRESSIVE, invasive, drastic or last-ditch surgical interventions, usually designed to save life but also potentially used to improve quality of life. The term suggests an emphasis on the attending surgeon, and some surgeons have been viewed by their contemporaries as heroes (in their medical or even their social contexts) in the past. Perhaps the most prominent examples in recent history include heart surgeons such as Christiaan Barnard (1922–2001; who conducted the first heart transplant operation) and Michael DeBakey (1908–2008; labelled the father of modern cardiovascular surgery, whose patients included Edward Duke of Windsor).

So why 'heroic patients'? Because until now, the patients who permitted audacious, pioneering or groundbreaking surgery to be carried out have tended to be sidelined in medical history, even though their contributions were indispensable. Further, collectively, they far outnumber the heroic surgeons. Barnard's 'achievement' would have been physically impossible without a heart to transplant, but the name 'Denise Darvall' (his unwitting donor; 1942–67) is not nearly so famous. His recipient patient, Louis Washkansky (1913–67), lived for less than 3 weeks after the operation, and Barnard was thousands of miles away at the time of his death.

Question 1: Why was Barnard not in attendance on Washkansky?

Heart transplant surgery was largely deemed a failure within 1 year of its introduction, and there was a virtual global moratorium on the procedure for the decade following. One American surgeon, Norman Shumway (1923–2006), continued to refine the technique, and prospects for the operation were renewed at the end of that decade (read about renal transplant failures in Section 7, Chapter 5, 'Transplantation'). Britain's official heart transplant programme began at Papworth Hospital in Cambridge in 1979.

Question 2: Who were Joe Burnside and Peter Everett?

Emergency!

Why is this relevant?

- Patient participation has always been central to the advancement of medical science, but patient consent has not always been sought as ethically as it is now.
- Medical definitions of success do not always involve protracted periods of survival among patients (who might therefore have different yardsticks by which to measure success, such as minimising pain or moderating the impact of treatments on their lifestyle).
- In the past, hundreds of people might have submitted to an operative procedure with little or no prospect of prolonged life, before that procedure was refined into the safe, successful 'routine' intervention of today.
- The introduction of routine clinical audit and publication of surgical mortality rates have helped to identify poorly performing hospitals and surgeons.

Further reading

Fox RC, Swazey JP. *The Courage to Fail: a social view of organ transplants and dialysis*. Chicago, IL: University of Chicago Press; 1974.

Stark T. *Knife to the Heart: the story of transplant surgery*. London: Macmillan; 1996.

2

War wounds and amputees

CONFLICT HAS HISTORICALLY BEEN AND CONTINUES TO BE A MAJOR cause of physical injury. This includes everything from a casual street fight between two antagonists to a pitched battle between opposing armies. Severe wounds, mangled limbs and loss of tissue are more likely to arise wherever opponents are armed. Battlefield surgery might have required the removal of an injured limb, whereby a surgeon would saw through muscle and bone. Amputation was one of the few major surgical interventions enjoying any prospect of patient survival prior to the introduction of anaesthesia and antisepsis for surgical procedures between 1840 and 1890. Approximately 30%–40% of amputees died, but that did at least leave 60%–70% alive. Coincidentally, people were not necessarily much better off away from the battle; planned surgery in an operating theatre probably carried a similar risk of infection.

The risk of post-operative infection meant that almost no operations were attempted on the chest or abdomen except as a last resort to save life or postpone death. Successful caesarean sections, for example, that preserved the lives of both mother and infant, were very rare before the late nineteenth century. Even so, some desperate interventions were surprisingly successful. Read an account of a mastectomy conducted in Paris in 1811 (written by Frances Burney [1752–1840], the woman who survived it), at www.mytimemachine.co.uk/operation.htm (accessed 19 April 2013).

Question 1: Aside from physical suffering, what in particular did Burney find emotionally distressing about the operation?

Question 2: How did her French doctors react to the procedure?

Burney was a novelist and playwright of some note, so she was perhaps ideally placed to provide this emotional and dramatic account. She lived for an impressive 29 years after the operation.

Not surprisingly, some patients refused to undergo surgery. For example, on 11 June 1828, a 31-year-old Scottish man was admitted to the Liverpool Infirmary with a fractured femur. One of the attending surgeons told the man that the break was so bad that it would be impossible to save his life without loss of limb. The man:

> would not be persuaded and said he would die with her [i.e. retaining his leg] and like a true north Briton stuck to his resolution in spite of the horrors of the judgement which Mr L [the surgeon] laid before him.
>
> Henry Peart, case notes 1827–1828, Wellcome Trust Library Ms 5263

The man died a week later on 18 June.

Why is this relevant?

- The context for patients presenting with injury changes from decade to decade, but the physical damage from injuries due to the events of wars and conflicts, such as bomb blasts, guns or knives, remains very similar.
- Acute pain and infection arising from surgical intervention were inevitabilities until relatively recently, as anaesthesia was not available for any procedures before the mid-1840s; however, surgery without benefit of pain relief still sometimes occurs in cut-off war zones.
- Fear of pain is a powerful motivating factor, now as then, and may lead people to make choices that contradict medical advice. An example of this is needle phobia, which is estimated to be experienced by 10% of the population.

Further reading

Snow SJ. *Blessed Days of Anaesthesia: how anaesthetics changed the world.* Oxford: Oxford University Press; 2008.

3

Road traffic accidents: from horse carriages to motor vehicles

FOR THE MAJOR PART OF HUMAN HISTORY, TRANSPORT ON LAND HAS comprised the horse for the prosperous or 'shanks' pony' (namely, walking) for the poor. Individual riders were unlikely to take any safety precautions such as wearing some form of helmet, and riding accidents were commonplace. Horse-drawn carriages were not necessarily any safer, although their coaching functions did extend the possibility of long-distance transport to those who could afford a ticket. Options proliferated in the 1820s, a decade which saw the introduction of both railways and buses, but danger from horses did not immediately decline.

In 1870, the *Cheshire Observer*, using annual data from the Accident Insurance Company, reported that in the previous year:

> [H]orse accidents predominated numbering as many as 339 and the compensations paid vary from £1.1s.6d to £500. Next is business accidents and here there are 192 examples of how men pursuing their ordinary occupations are liable to the contingency of disablement...
>
> News, Accident Insurance, *Cheshire Observer*, 26 August 1871: 3

Ten years later, horse accidents still dominated the accident-related statistics. This is illustrated by the following address on 'The number of deaths from negligence, violence and misadventure in the UK' made by Cornelius Walford (1827–85) to the Statistical Society in 1880: 'Railways were by no means the cause of the greatest annual number of violent deaths, for more persons were yearly killed by horses and horse carriage accidents than by all the railways of the kingdom' (News, The Statistical Society, *Morning Post*, 17 February 1881: 3).

Horse-drawn omnibuses were introduced to London in 1829 by George Shillibeer (1797–1866), who launched 22-seater buses drawn by three horses. Tickets were a third of the price of traditional horse-drawn carriages, so this became a popular form of transport. However, accidents occurred – one such incident happened in 1867 at St Helens and involved 30 workmen returning from their annual trip to Liverpool. According to a witness, the omnibus lost control descending a hill because one of the horses became restive. Those travelling on the outside of the vehicle all sustained bad injuries and two men died. Notwithstanding such tragic accidents and in spite of the ubiquity of rail travel, there were almost 4000 horse omnibuses operating in London by the turn of the twentieth century.

The motor vehicle would have been a presence on British roads long before then had it not been for The Locomotive Act (or 'Red Flag Act') of 1865. This required self-propelled vehicles to be preceded by a man walking in front of the vehicle waving a red flag and prohibited travelling at speeds greater than 2 mph in towns. At that time, such vehicles were heavy steam-powered road 'locomotives', which, due to their weight, caused damage to the highways; their speed also triggered public safety concerns. When the act was eventually repealed, cars proliferated, giving rise to even more concerns about safety.

In 1917, the London 'Safety First' Council (later called the Royal Society for the Prevention of Accidents [RoSPA]) was established in response to the alarming number of accidental deaths on the roads due to the black outs of the First World War. The London 'Safety First' Council's pamphlet and poster entitled *Hints to Drivers of Horsed and Motor Vehicles, and to Cyclists* pointed out that in London in 1916 over 46 000 people had been involved in avoidable road accidents, 833 of whom died. The council successfully campaigned for pedestrians to walk in the opposite direction from traffic, which led to a 70% reduction in deaths over 1 year. During the next 30 years, the RoSPA was responsible for public education campaigns to improve safety, both on the roads and in the workplace, and lobbied for several improvements such as recognisable road crossing places, better street lighting, the licensing of all drivers and the introduction of a highway code, which came into existence in 1931. The RoSPA conducted useful research that revealed the peak danger ages for child pedestrians (7 years), cyclists (14 to 16 years) and motorists (21 to 26 years). It subsequently held its first National Children's Safety Week in 1950 and turned its cycle training into a National Child Cycling Proficiency Scheme. By 1974, child cycling fatalities in Britain had been reduced to less than 100 per year for the first time. More recently, the society campaigned successfully for legislation on drink-driving, compulsory seatbelts and prohibition of handheld mobile phones while driving.

Question 1: When did this legislation occur?

Question 2: What form of transport causes a disproportionate number of road traffic accidents in Britain?

Why is this relevant?

- Travel, by whatever means, entails risk. Although horse-related accidents are today responsible for far fewer deaths than in the nineteenth century, those that do occur frequently result in injuries that require hospital treatment and tend to involve serious head or spinal damage.
- Safety campaigners have been very successful in highlighting to individuals

how to mitigate risk. Without their work, our roads would have continued to kill or injure vast numbers of people, leading to heavy social and health costs.

- Nevertheless, there is often a balance to be achieved between safety legislation and individual autonomy. The RoSPA has been often accused of being a killjoy, despite it advocating sensible rather than extreme safety measures.

Further reading

Lee CE. *The Horse Bus as a Vehicle.* London: British Transport Commission; 1962.

Royal Society for the Prevention of Accidents (RoSPA). *History of the Royal Society for the Prevention of Accidents.* Available at: www.rospa.com/about/history/default.aspx (accessed 20 April 2013).

4

Accidents in the workplace

ACCIDENTS IN THE WORKPLACE WERE A MAJOR SOURCE OF MORBIDITY and mortality in the nineteenth century with the advent of the crowded working conditions typical of industrialising countries. The history of social and occupational health medicine largely reflects the history of industry and labour from the industrial era. However, in pre-industrial times, some important publications drew attention to the link between working environment, disease and accidents. For example, in 1526, Georg Bauer (1494–1555), a German mineralogist, wrote extensively in his book *De Re Metallica* [On the nature of metals] about the diseases and accidents common among miners and offered recommendations on their prevention. Bernardo Ramazzini (1633–1714) published the first most comprehensive book on occupational morbidity in 1713, *De Morbis Artificum Diatriba* [The diseases of workers].

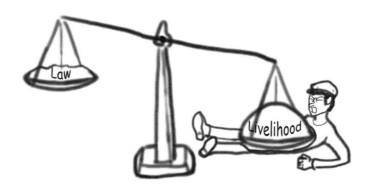

The Lot of the Sawgrinder

In 1843, Dr G Calvert Holland published *The Vital Statistics of Sheffield*, in which he commented on how saw-grinders were 'peculiarly liable to accidents from the breaking of stone and from becoming entangled in machinery. 42 deceased since 1821 and 78 accidents'. His terse descriptions conceal the inevitable emotional and functional impact of such accidents: 'Case 1: lame for breaking stone;

Case 2: arm broke, entangled in machinery; Case 3: skull severely fractured; Case 4: leg broken, now a cripple.'

Question 1: What effects did such injuries have on families?

Mining was another dangerous occupation. Between 1850 and 1914, 90 000 entries of death or injury were listed in the Mines Inspectorate's reports. This inspectorate was first formed in 1843, 10 years after the first inspectorate for factories had been established to prevent overworking of child textile workers (*see* Section 4, Chapter 7, 'Child welfare'). A year later, in 1844, the first legislation in Britain was passed to ensure that factory employees were kept safe from dangerous machinery.

Unfortunately, despite the presence of the inspectorates, much of the legislation proved difficult to enforce. This is illustrated by the lack of efficacy of several chimney sweeps acts passed throughout the nineteenth century; these amounted to tokenism until all sweeps were licensed and the police empowered to enforce the law. Of course, there were some nineteenth-century employers who had socialist ideals and high ethical principles, such as the Quaker Cadbury brothers and Robert Owen (1771–1858), but employers were more likely to be persuaded by economic arguments for consolidating what we would now describe as 'occupational health and safety'. Although the first law in Britain requiring an employer to provide compensation to a worker involved in an accident was not passed until 1906 (whereas such legislation – the Employers' Liability Law – was introduced in Prussia in 1884 by Chancellor Otto von Bismarck, although the reasons for this were political rather than altruistic), some employers realised that preventing injury in the workforce was more cost-effective than loosing skilled workers and endangering morale. The medical costs were high, too. The records of one British voluntary hospital, North Ormesby in Yorkshire, show that between 1883 and 1908 the majority of admissions were of male manual employees in heavy industries (such as railways and ironworks) who presented with fractures or burns due to accidents at work.

The twentieth century saw a shift of attitude with regard to the balance of employer and worker responsibility for injury at work, which increasingly became enshrined by legislative change. While, in the nineteenth century, the risk of injury was generally seen as one of the acceptable risks of working and receiving a wage, in the twentieth century, workplace injury became a social problem that could only be addressed by government intervention. Organisations such as the London 'Safety First' Council played a key role in a number of ways – for example, by setting up an industrial committee in 1917, appointing safety engineers to advise industrial members in workplaces on accident prevention and running several safety campaigns. Further legislation was then passed between the early part of the twentieth century and the Health and Safety at Work Act etc. in 1974, which improved health and safety in the agricultural and nuclear industries.

Question 2: What did the Health and Safety at Work Act etc. 1974 do?

Since the Health and Safety in the Workplace Act etc. 1974, accident prevention has spilled over into almost every area and location of human activity, from do-it-yourself work around the home to using bouncy castles. Many people feel frustrated and irritated at this intrusion of the state into their lives – as the headlines of two articles attest: 'Park benches removed in Crawley after 'absurd' health and safety ruling' (*The Argus*, 6 September 2012) and 'Councillor's frustration as health and safety stops offenders from carrying out community service' (S. Crowther, STV Aberdeen City [website], 13 October 2011). Yet, in those countries with little or struggling health and safety legislation, poor working conditions continue to lead to significant mortality rates, as an article titled 'China coal mine deaths fall "but still remain high"' in the *China Daily* highlights: '2,433 people died in coal mine accidents last year, 198 fewer than in 2009' (W. Huazhong, 26 February 2011, 1). Although China has tried to prioritise working standards for its mining employees in recent years, it still has a mortality rate which is at least ten times higher than that of developed countries (average for developed countries is 0.02 deaths per million tons of coal production).

Why is this relevant?

- Without the reform movement of the nineteenth century, it would have been unlikely that improvements in British working conditions would have occurred to the extent that they have.
- Casualty departments within the NHS deal with accidents daily. Their capacity would need to be much greater if there were not effective health and safety legislation.
- There is a tension between what is perceived as state over-intervention and protection of the vulnerable. The headline from the *China Daily* demonstrates what happens when there is little enforceable legislation, but the British news items tacitly argue that legislation can defeat common sense.

Further reading

Abrams HK. A short history of occupational health. *Journal of Public Health Policy*. 2001; **22**(1): 34–80.

Mill C. *Regulating Health and Safety in the British Mining Industry, 1800–1914*. Farnham: Ashgate; 2010.

Warren MD, compiler. *A Chronology of State Medicine, Public Health, Welfare and Related Services in Britain 1066–1999*. London: Faculty of Public Health Medicine, Royal Colleges of Physicians of the United Kingdom; 2000. Available at: www.fph.org.uk/uploads/r_chronology_of_state_medicine.pdf (accessed 24 November 2012).

www.cmhrc.co.uk

5

Primary care begins at home

ILLNESS AND ACCIDENTS DEMANDING AN IMMEDIATE RESPONSE HAVE always received their first intervention from the people closest to hand. In public places in the modern age, such as at the theatre, emergencies often provoke the question 'Is there a doctor in the house?' and most medical students are taught early in their training the skills of life support. Yet, most sudden illnesses and accidents in history have occurred when there is no formal practitioner at hand, at home or at work. Relatives, friends and colleagues have comprised the source of earliest medical help, thus untrained understandings of human bodies, and of possible remedies or treatments, have been central to the experience of primary care.

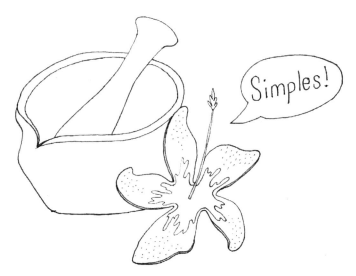

Medical texts were among the first books to be produced with the advent of printing but, in a largely illiterate society, herbal folklore was transmitted via word of mouth and learned by domestic practice. Plants found in gardens, cultivated as crops or scattered in hedges and verges, might be dried, ground, mixed with liquid or foods for topical, oral or anal administration. Substances taken on their own were known as 'simples' because they did not require elaborate recipes or any equipment in their manufacture. Leonard Sowerby's *Ladies' Dispensatory*

of 1652 listed a range of different options for each type of complaint. Simples recommended for healing wounds included elm leaves, sycamore gum and basil seed. More complicated mixtures, or 'compounds', obviously took longer to prepare but could remain an attractive option in contexts where the cost of trained advice and medicines might be beyond a family's reach.

> **Question**: How would the use of ground ivy in the treatment of coughs and mild lung complaints be regarded in the present day – as harmful, futile, remotely helpful or actively advisable?

Home care and cure was the province of adult women in most families. One such woman was Elizabeth Isham (1609–54), a gentlewoman of seventeenth-century Northamptonshire. We know about Isham because she left a book of remembrance and a receipt book, providing evidence that she learned domestic medical practice from other women in her family. Her great-grandmother was described as 'skilful in surgery' while other entries suggest she learned or copied remedies from her aunt. Isham used family know-how and advice from neighbours in conjunction with herbals and gardening books to inform her lay practice.

As literacy became more widespread, printed 'self-help' manuals became viable. Nicholas Culpeper's (1616–54) *Complete Herbal* of 1653 supplied information to the reading public that had previously been available only to those educated few who could read Latin. This brought him into conflict with both the Royal College of Physicians and the Society of Apothecaries for challenging their monopolies of medical knowledge. Less controversial was William Buchan's (1729–1805) *Domestic Medicine*, which was first published in 1769, ran to over 20 editions and was one of the most popular books of the later eighteenth century (*see* Section 8, Chapter 1, 'From spicer to pharmacist').

Why is this relevant?

- Cultural and family practice, traditions and understandings of health and illness are embedded in patient experiences, thus modify illness behaviour.
- Women have long held primary care-giving roles and, despite the erosion of gender stereotyping characteristic of the developed world, women may still regard family health as their province and speciality.
- Some traditional, herbal and folk medicine may have been misguided or harmful, but some age-old remedies provide the basis for viable chemical treatments and/or are useful in palliative medicine. Can you think of some examples?

Further reading

Balaban C, Erlan J, Siderits R, editors. *The Ladies' Dispensatory*. Sowerby L, author. New York, NY: Routledge; 2002.

6

Fatality, the Coroner's Court and medical responsibility

SUDDEN, UNNATURAL AND VIOLENT DEATHS HAVE BEEN OF INTEREST to human beings from the earliest recorded times and, in Britain, this concern gave rise to the inquisition post-mortem, overseen by a coroner, from 1194. In other words, coroners have the longest-established title of all the other professions you are likely to encounter in a medical career. Historically, though, coroners were not medically trained. It was only in the twentieth century that medical expertise was found essential for the exercise of coronial authority. Before the late nineteenth century, coroners were frequently lawyers (and de facto politicians, in as much as the post was usually elected).

Historical inquests empanelled a jury of at least 12 people who literally viewed the body of the deceased and tried to reach a verdict about a cause of death. Anyone with knowledge of the death was asked to present themselves; if they failed to do so, the coroner could summon them on pain of contempt. Medical witnesses could be called to give evidence about the physical demeanour of a cadaver, with a view to determining the cause of death. The involvement of medical men and women was most pertinent when clues as to the cause of death were subtle, as in cases of smothering or narcotic poison, and an autopsy or other investigations might be ordered.

However, medical witnesses could find themselves in difficulty if their testimony or that of others at the inquest indicated that neglect of medical duty, medical error or any other form of practitioner-related harm contributed to the person's death. Doctors, midwives and practitioners of all kinds could be deemed personally liable, and they could be most vulnerable to criticism when they were employed on a contractual basis to serve an arm of local government. The English Poor Law (or Public Assistance as it was renamed from 1929) was a form of welfare in existence in Britain before the NHS, and employed many practitioners, nurses, midwives and others to attend those too poor to employ medical personnel on their own behalf. Such people could be both overworked and quite isolated in an era before organised representation was available. In other words, there is a long history of over-stretched staffing in British state medicine and an established tendency to apportion blame if things go wrong.

Emergency!

> **Question**: What organisations exist in the twenty-first century to support and advise medical professionals accused of negligence?

In 1862, Frederick Robinson, a surgeon, was one of the district medical officers of the Stepney Poor Law Union in London. He was asked to attend the delivery of a poor woman, Elizabeth Cruse, but this was not to prove an instance of straightforward childbirth. Cruse died, and the subsequent inquest found Robinson guilty of her manslaughter. Robinson's trial at the Old Bailey and subsequent conviction was widely reported in the press and became something of a cause célèbre. The punishment was just 4 months in prison, but Robinson could not hope to practice in Britain after his release. He sailed to Australia in 1863 and practised until his death in New Zealand in 1869.

On the establishment of the NHS in 1948, the state became responsible for injuries caused by NHS staff other than doctors. As such, doctors were required to continue to be members of one of the medical insurance schemes, such as the Medical Defence Union or Medical Protection Society, for their NHS practice as well as for any private practice they undertook. However, the state's responsibility was limited by the principle of 'Crown indemnity', which meant that the Crown (and by extension the NHS as an agent of the Crown) could not be litigated against. In 1995, Crown indemnity was abolished and healthcare trusts were obliged to shoulder the risk of claims for compensation for acts of negligence carried out by their staff. Trusts agreed to extend their responsibility to directly employed hospital doctors with regard to their NHS work. Doctors remained individually responsible for their private clinical practice. The cost for trusts and individual doctors has risen remorselessly and has led to calls to limit compensation payments.

As far as we are aware, there has been very little historical research on the shifts in medico-legal responsibility between the era of Robinson's conviction and the time of writing this book. Much remains to be understood about the relationship in the past between the laws in the statute books and the development of case law in this area as well as about the changing understandings of medical duty.

Medical professionals may still choose to take out personal insurance for a number of reasons. They may wish to be covered for work they undertake privately (so, outside the remit of the NHS trusts) or specifically to tackle differences of opinion they have individually with their own trust/employer.

Why is this relevant?

- Coroners use medicine and law to determine causes of death in the present, but they embody an ancient tradition.
- The public nature of an inquest is historic and justified by the desire to obtain as much information as possible about sudden and violent deaths; however, this can now, as in the past, have unintended consequences for witnesses and other participants.
- The actions of medical professionals have always been subject to potential

misunderstanding and challenge; this is not solely a phenomenon of modern life.

Further reading

Price K. "Where is the fault": the starvation of Edward Cooper at the Isle of Wight workhouse in 1877. *Social History of Medicine*. 2012; 26:1: 21–37.

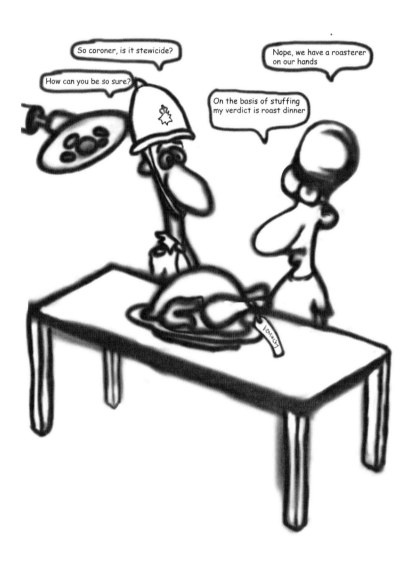

7

The history of resuscitation in England

THE ROYAL HUMANE SOCIETY WAS FOUNDED IN 1774 TO REVIVE PEOPLE who had seemingly drowned. Death by drowning was common in a society in which people did not often swim for leisure. It was modelled on a similar institution founded in Amsterdam in 1767 (where many accidental deaths involved falls into canals). The foundation of the English society was also motivated by a desire to prevent premature burials. In eighteenth-century England, there was considerable fear about the prospect of being buried alive (and the terrors attendant on then dying of suffocation while entombed). Some people even stipulated in their will that there should be a long delay between their death and their burial, or that one of their arteries be severed after 'death' to prevent any revival.

The society offered advice on how to resuscitate the drowned, suffocated or comatose. With the benefit of hindsight, it is possible for us to identify those historical strategies likely to promote health, or at least do no additional harm (such as gently warming victims) as well as measures that were at best idiosyncratic and at worst harmful nonsense.

> **Question**: Can you find examples of some of the more outlandish methods for bringing people back to life?

Naturally, a combination of trial and error, news of successes and failures elsewhere (after similar societies were established in Europe and America) and the gradual advancement of medical science, contributed to increasing success for the society's advocates. It is telling that the society no longer supplies information on the means of resuscitation, owing to the increasing risk of being sued should advice be misapplied. In a litigious twenty-first century context, it is perhaps wiser to reward the saving of life without necessarily prescribing methods for doing so.

It took rather longer for medical practitioners to accept resuscitation as a legitimate technique. The first known case in which a medical doctor used external chest compressions to achieve human resuscitation took place in 1903. Defibrillators have been used since the 1950s. Modern cardiopulmonary resuscitation was developed from the 1960s onwards but continues to be refined in the 2000s. In 2008, the American Heart Association, for example, recommended that chest compression need not be accompanied by artificial respiration but may comprise a hands-only response.

Why is this relevant?

- Resuscitation is a relatively recent addition to professional (as opposed to lay) medical practice.
- Medical scientific ability has now exceeded some people's expectations; on some occasions, resuscitation is possible but no longer desirable, hence the ability to be able to request a do-not-resuscitate order.
- Other people fear that they will not be revived simply because they are older, a campaign issue for the organisation Age Concern. In addition, there is a concern among some of the public that unscrupulous or impatient health teams might fail to revive a vegetative patient so that their organs might be used more swiftly for transplantation. In the eventuality that this is the case, some staff may feel pressured into complicity or obliged to become whistle-blowers.
- Since the risks surrounding resuscitation are so evident, there is an increasing divide between medicine and the preferences of kin. Hospitals, doctors, pharmacists and other medical staff are concerned about litigation, while families may perceive medical teams as cruel (either because they terminate life or because they do not).

Further reading

Royal Humane Society. *The History of the Society*. Available at: www.royalhumanesociety.org.uk/html/history.html (accessed 19 April 2013).

From war to shell shock to post-traumatic stress disorder

FOUR HUNDRED YEARS BEFORE POST-TRAUMATIC STRESS DISORDER (PTSD) was classified as a psychiatric disorder, William Shakespeare gave us a pretty accurate description of the main symptoms in *Henry IV, Part 1*. In the second act, Hotspur's wife, Kate, complains about her husband's regular involvement in potentially mortal combat and his consequent odd behaviour:

> O, my good lord, why are you thus alone?
> For what offence have I this fortnight been
> A banish'd woman from my Harry's bed?
> Tell me, sweet lord, what is't that takes from thee
> Thy stomach, pleasure and thy golden sleep?
> Why dost thou bend thine eyes upon the earth,
> And start so often when thou sit'st alone?
> Why hast thou lost the fresh blood in thy cheeks;
> And given my treasures and my rights of thee
> To thick-eyed musing and curst melancholy?
> In thy faint slumbers I by thee have watch'd,
> And heard thee murmur tales of iron wars;
> Speak terms of manage [horsemanship] to thy bounding steed;
> Cry 'Courage! to the field!' And thou hast talk'd
> Of sallies and retires, of trenches, tents,
> Of palisadoes, frontiers, parapets,
> Of basilisks, of cannon, culverin,
> Of prisoners' ransom and of soldiers slain,
> And all the currents of a heady fight.
> Thy spirit within thee hath been so at war,
> And thus hath so bestirr'd thee in thy sleep,
> That beads of sweat have stood upon thy brow
> Like bubbles in a late-disturbed stream;
> And in thy face strange motions have appear'd,
> Such as we see when men restrain their breath

On some great sudden hest. O, what portents are these?
Some heavy business hath my lord in hand,
And I must know it, else he loves me not.

Henry IV, Part 1, Act 2, Scene 3, lines 895–923

Question 1: What diagnostic symptoms of PTSD can you identify in this speech?

In this scene, Kate identifies changes in her husband's behaviour which she attributes to his experiences of battle. During the First World War, the term 'shellshock' was coined to describe a diverse group of conditions which appeared to develop after combat. These ranged from what we would now call anxiety states to hysterical conversion disorders. Although PTSD and shellshock clearly overlap, they are not the same condition. They both require exposure to an event perceived as 'exceptionally threatening or catastrophic' but for shellshock this is specifically battle exposure, whereas a wide range of events may act as precipitants of PTSD, such as the experience of being mugged, sexually assaulted or of a road traffic accident.

Before the First World War, military doctors might have gone as far as diagnosing 'exhaustion' following the stress of battle but nervous breakdown due to the horrors of war was not an acknowledged condition. Therefore, the number of casualties suffering from shell shock, who presented with a bizarre range of physical and mental disabilities during the war, took the army by surprise. Shell shock was particularly alarming because officers were twice as likely to be affected as men in the ranks, and this had a seriously deleterious effect on morale and discipline. By the end of the war, some 80 000 soldiers had experienced a mental breakdown. This statistic may be an underestimate because those soldiers with hysterical symptoms such as aphonia were often mistakenly diagnosed with an organic disease and sent to medical wards. Further, because of stigma, medical officers often preferred to label soldiers as being 'sick' or having 'debility' rather than having a mental condition.

Initially, the pathological mechanism for shell shock was thought to be physical damage from exploding shells, but this became less likely when it emerged that shell shock also occurred in those who had not been directly exposed to shell blast. Another popular theory was that victims had 'tainted' heredities, an idea in keeping with the popular theory of degeneration (*see* Section 2, Chapter 4, 'Friend or foe?'). However, since most shell shock victims were officers and therefore considered to represent 'England's finest blood', this theory was dismissed as a 'slur on the noblest of our race'. Shell shock presented in two distinct ways. Officers tended to be diagnosed with neurasthenia (akin to a chronic anxiety state) whereas men in the ranks – that is, from the lower or working class – were more often thought to present with an acute hysterical disorder. Before the war, both these diagnoses were treated dismissively by neurologists and asylum doctors; in particular, those with hysterical symptoms were considered malingerers.

Emergency!

The military response during the war was similar. Some medical board neurologists took the view that when no organic disorder was identifiable, the patient must be faking symptoms. Many military men were appalled at the concept of 'shell shock', with responses ranging from, 'a respectable name for fear' through to 'the idea and name . . . is a devastating menace'. This was in stark contrast to the public, parliamentary and newspaper response, which was very sympathetic.

Treatment methods varied depending on aetiological beliefs. One apparently successful approach was the use of suggestion in combination with aversive interventions such as electrical faradisation. This particular treatment had been pioneered by a Canadian-born therapist, Lewis Yealland (1884–1951), at Aldershot and became a popular method for treating hysterical shell shock. Aphonia, for example, was treated by applying electrical shocks to the larynx until the patient screamed, whereupon he was deemed cured! However, the cure only lasted until the patient's next exposure to gun fire. A number of other doctors, particularly those working at Maghull, used psychotherapeutic methods – in particular, abreactive techniques – to help patients relive painful emotional memories, which were considered to have been repressed. This approach drew on Freudian theory, which was still very unpopular with the British medical establishment. Nevertheless, many army neurologists were more inclined to accept a psychodynamic conceptualisation of shellshock after encountering a paper, *The Repression of War Experience* delivered by a neurologist, Captain WH Rivers (1864–1922), to the Royal Society of Medicine in 1917 and published in the *Lancet* the following year. In this paper, Rivers embraced some of Freud's ideas but dismissed a more contentious area, that is the importance of repressed infantile sexual impulses. His conceptualisation of shellshock was as a psychological condition precipitated by a conflict between fear and duty on the battlefield. After leaving Maghull, Rivers worked at Craiglockhart War Hospital where his most famous patients were the poets Siegfried Sassoon and Wilfred Owen.

> **Question 2**: There were a number of other pioneers of medical psychology and psychotherapeutic approaches. Who were these people and where did they practice?

Why is this relevant?

- Shell shock helped to bring mental illness into the public's awareness and show that anyone was at risk of developing a mental illness, including those deserving of military honours.
- Because there were so many ex-servicemen requiring treatment and pensions after the war, shell shock facilitated the development of a more modern approach to the care of the mentally ill. With the passing of the Mental Treatment Act 1930, psychotherapeutic treatments and outpatient clinics were increasingly developed.
- The British Army now recognises and manages PTSD resulting from combat much better than it did in the past. Recent research, (Sundin J *et al.*, 2011)

revealed that its prevalence in the army has remained low (1.6%–6.0%) and stable for the last 6 years, although the rate of alcohol misuse has risen in that time to 20%. In contrast, another recent paper (Reed R *et al.*, 2012) highlighted that PTSD is often under-diagnosed in the general population.

Further reading

Barker P. Regeneration. *The Regeneration Trilogy* [novels]. London: Penguin; 2008.

Barker P. The Eye in the Door. London: Penguin; 2008.

Barker P. The Ghost Road. London: Penguin; 2012.

Bennett G. Shakespeare and post-traumatic stress disorder – extra. *British Journal of Psychiatry*. 2011; **198**: 255.

Howorth PW. The treatment of shell-shock: cognitive therapy before its time. *The Psychiatrist*. 2000; **24**: 225–7.

Reed R, Fazel M, Goldring L. Easily Missed? Post traumatic stress disorder. *British Medical Journal*. 2012; **344**: e3790.

Sassoon S. *The War Poems of Siegfried Sassoon*. London: Faber and Faber; 1983.

Stone M. Shellshock and the psychologists. In: Bynum WF, Porter R, Shepherd M, editors. *The Anatomy of Madness*. Vol. 2, *Institutions and society*. London and New York, NY: Tavistock; 1985. pp. 242–71.

Sundin J, Forbes H, Fear NT *et al*. The impacts of the conflicts of Iraq and Afghanistan. *Int. Review of Psychiatry*. 2011; **23**: 153–9.

Section 2

The pleasures of life: food, drink, drugs and sex

1

Fagged out: the medical uses and abuses of tobacco

TOBACCO WAS IMPORTED TO EUROPE FROM THE NEW WORLD (especially from Virginia) from around 1600. The leaves were smoked in pipes, chewed or inhaled (as snuff), and tobacco consumption became particularly popular in England and The Netherlands. Men and women, rich and poor, enjoyed the new commodity. Cigarettes and cigars came into use in the nineteenth century.

Early medical enthusiasts included Nicholas Culpeper (1616–54), an apothecary with a clear addiction to pipe smoking. Tobacco was credited with clearing the head and aiding digestion, but it was also prescribed in the form of an enema as a laxative. It did have its early critics, but on moral rather than medical grounds. No less a person than King James I and VI of England and Scotland, respectively, actually published a treatise opposed to tobacco consumption. It was not until the later eighteenth century that there was any suggestion of harmful consequences of tobacco use. John Hill (1716–75) was the author of a 26-volume work entitled *The Vegetable System* and he observed a link between the practice of frequent recourse to snuff (a elite fashionable affectation during the eighteenth century) and cancer of the nose. Austin Bradford Hill and Richard Doll were the first modern scientists to demonstrate the causal link between smoking tobacco and contracting lung cancer in research published over 1950–54 using randomised clinical trials; however, it was not until 1996 that litigants successfully sued the global tobacco industry on the grounds of the carcinogenic properties of tobacco.

> **Question**: The first lawsuits were brought against tobacco companies in 1954; why did it take so long for any the plaintiffs in these sorts of cases to achieve success? What did Adolf Hitler have to do with it?

The cultural impact of tobacco and, specifically, cigarettes was immense in the twentieth century. Hollywood actors were encouraged or required to smoke on screen, with some film action and plots hinging on the business of acquiring or lighting cigarettes. Poignantly, the actor Humphrey Bogart, who frequently sported a lit cigarette in photographic portraits, died from cancer of the oesophagus aged

57 years old. Latterly, there has been an ironic interest in the continued survival of the tobacco industry; see, for instance, director Jason Reitman's film *Thank You For Smoking* (2005).

Why is this relevant?

- People embark on tobacco use for social purposes or owing to cultural pressures but maintain it by reason of addiction.
- Patients present with a variety of complaints directly or indirectly attributable to smoking, but the extent to which they can be identified as the 'saboteurs' of their own good health is questionable.
- Approximately half of all tobacco users will go on to die from a (preventable) tobacco-related complaint.

Further reading

Daynard RA, Bates C, Francey N. Tobacco litigation worldwide. *British Medical Journal*. 2000; **32**(7227): 111–13.

2

Sweet teeth: the history of sugar consumption

TOOTH DECAY ARISES FROM THE RANGE OF CHEMICAL CHALLENGES posed to human dentition by dietary intake. In the modern world, acids and sugars, particularly those lurking quietly in processed foodstuffs and drinks, can have a devastating effect on tooth enamel. Consequently, an industry has arisen to help us combat decay, plaque and build-up of scale on teeth via toothpastes, brushes, flosses and mouthwashes alongside the intervention of dental practitioners. However, people have not always had access to resources for dental hygiene.

Natural sugars such as fructose and lactose are a frequent and recurring presence in the omnivorous human diet; refined sugars, treacles and other sweet products are a relatively recent addition. Sugarcane grows most successfully in hot tropical climates, thus sugar was not a product routinely available in European markets until the development of transatlantic trade. Therefore, sugar was a luxury commodity in the sixteenth and seventeenth centuries. By 1800, it was produced and shipped in very large quantities, which drove down the price and made it increasingly available to ordinary people. Treacle akin to molasses was even purchased for the inhabitants of English workhouses in the eighteenth century, to add savour to porridges and other bland dishes.

A visible and bodily consequence of sugar's widespread availability was the decay of teeth, first among the richer members of society who could afford the derivatives of sugar such as treacle and later among working people. The causes of enamel erosion were not widely or well understood, so the first responses to tooth decay were reactive rather than prophylactic: bad teeth were pulled out, without benefit of pain relief. As a consequence, it was quite common for people to become toothless well before old age.

> **Question**: How might sets of false teeth have been manufactured? What range of materials was available prior to the advent of modern plastics and chemical industries?

Toothbrushes and powders had been developed by the end of the eighteenth century, supplying a means of dental hygiene to those who could afford it (and who remained conscientious). According to newspaper advertisements of the 1790s, ordinary brushes could be purchased for three to six pence each, but a superior brush might be had for nine pence or one shilling. However, early brushes suffered from problems of durability, as the brush fibres tended to come loose in people's mouths. Thus, some people were clearly willing to invest in sensible and potentially antibacterial activity well before the development of germ theory (*see* Section 4, Chapter 4, 'The germ theory of disease').

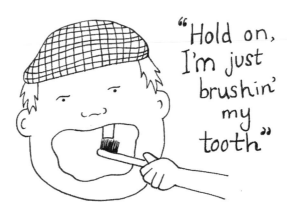

The discomforts of dental ill-health and the pain of tooth pulling encouraged a brisk market in alleged alternative treatments, in which untrained individuals offered salves and other applications and made stout claims of efficacy. The sellers may genuinely have believed in their nostrums (and if they contained opiate derivatives, they may well have performed some pain-killing function), but they may equally have exploited patients' hopes and fears to peddle ineffective or actively harmful substances. In this sense, dentistry and medicine alike were subject to professional challenges from untrained or unscrupulous rivals.

Dentistry as a profession (as opposed to a marketplace service of tooth pulling) became codified by the Dentists Act 1878, which ensured that everyone who wanted to call themselves a 'dentist' first had to serve an apprenticeship, take a preliminary examination and pursue study at both a dental hospital and a general hospital before sitting a final examination. A Staffordshire dentist, Arnold Wain, enjoyed a career in the Potteries spanning from 1910 to 1959. For the majority of that time, his work was largely characterised by the need to remove teeth and fit dentures rather than perform fillings or other repair work.

Why is this relevant?

- A focus on diet, obesity and heart disease by policymakers and health professionals in the modern, first world can mask the continued problem of tooth decay.
- Difficulties of accessing dental care through the NHS following the govern-

ment's reforms of 2006 and the increasing cost of private work have led to some deterioration in British dental health.

- In the developing world, there is a medical and dental marketplace that is relatively unregulated. Such circumstances, just like in the eighteenth century, favour the proliferation of inadequately trained practitioners who are able to offer very competitive fees. Low prices together with cheap fares and Internet advertising have led to significant medical and dental tourism. This has led the British Dental Association to express concern that more and more patients with complications are presenting following treatments abroad.

Further reading

Harrison C. Arnold Wain, dentist: a case study of dental care provision in the Staffordshire Potteries, 1910–1959. *Staffordshire Studies.* 1996; **8**: 96–111.

Jones C. French dentists and English teeth in the long eighteenth century: a tale of two cities and one dentist. In: Bivens R, Pickstone JV, editors. *Medicine, Madness and Social History: essays in honour of Roy Porter.* Basingstoke: Palgrave; 2007. pp. 73–89.

Shammas C. *The Pre-Industrial Consumer in England and America.* Oxford: Oxford University Press; 1990.

Welshman J. Dental health as a neglected issue in medical history: the school dental service in England and Wales, 1900–40. *Medical History.* 1998; **42**(3): 306–27.

3

Alcohol: master or servant?

[A]lcohol has existed longer than all human memory. It has outlived genera-tions, nations, epochs and ages. It is part of us and that is fortunate indeed. For although alcohol will always be the master of some, for most of us it will continue to be the servant of man . . .

Morris E. Chafetz, founding director of the National Institute of Alcohol Abuse and Alcoholism, from *Liquor:The Servant of Man.* Boston: Little Brown and Co; 1965: 223

The health and social costs of immoderate drinking have led to growing political and societal disquiet about the accessibility of alcohol today, which the media likes to highlight: 'Our biggest drug problem is an ocean of cheap alcohol', for example, is the title of an article by John Harris in *The Guardian* of 26 July 2007. Concerns have not changed in the intervening years: 'BOOZE fuelled Brits spilled onto streets . . .' reported *The Sun*'s staff reporter on January 2, 2013. The head-line was followed by several uncomplimentary photographs of drunk, uninhibited young men and women.

Alcohol has fulfilled several roles in human societies such as:
- a source of calories
- an analgesic
- an antiseptic
- a medical agent such as a digestive or hypnotic
- a social lubricant
- a source of pleasure – for 'bringing joy to God and Man' (Judges 9:13).

Consequently, alcohol has been highly valued and used across cultures through-out history. It has also been an important component of religious rituals. The Egyptians, who worshipped Osiris as their god of wine and credited him with inventing beer, used alcohol for funerary purposes, leaving some in the tombs of the pharaohs for their use in the afterlife. Many religious faiths use wine sac-ramentally. For example, wine plays a mystical role in the Eucharist of Catholic services while, within Jewish practice, the end of the Sabbath is marked by wine being passed around the whole family including the children (the ritual is called the 'Kiddush'). The good health of the Jews was attributed historically to their moderate use of alcohol and exposure to it at an early age. Religious texts like the New and Old Testaments, the Talmud and the Koran do, however, contain inconsistencies regarding the place of alcohol, which suggests that religious attitudes were equivocal, although all discourage excessive drinking. Such texts are open to subjective interpretation, so practice tends to reflect current cultural attitudes. This might explain why Islamic views have become less relaxed in recent times – although not ubiquitously, as suggested by the recent news story 'A drinkers guide to Islam: a Palestinian beerfest is not as bizarre as it seems' (K Diab, *The Guardian*, 8 October 2011), which concerned a small remote village on the West Bank that has its own brewery where Muslims congregate to drink.

Attitudes towards alcohol use have been influenced in the last 100 years by an appreciation of the deleterious health effects of chronic use. Until the early twentieth century, a medical distinction existed between fermented drinks such as wine, cider and beer, which were considered 'hygienic', and distilled drinks. Indeed, beer was much safer to drink than water before public sanitation became properly established in the mid to late nineteenth century. This is because water had to be boiled in the process of beer production, which helped to kill off most germs, and because alcohol acts as an antiseptic. For centuries, people had been used to drinking 'small beer' rather than water because its very low alcohol content made the water safer. However, in the mind of the public and, indeed, those of many doctors, distilled drinks caused alcoholism. This belief was only challenged during the First World War when the male population of France was comprehensively medically examined for the first time. It was found that organ damage was as prevalent in wine drinkers as it was in those who drank spirits. By the 1920s, it was well established that it was the amount rather than the type of alcohol consumed that was the cause of a number of medical problems. In 1937, Elvin Morton Jellineck (1890–1963), an American physician, founded the Research Council on the Problems of Alcohol and classified the medical consequences of chronic alcoholism. His definition of alcoholism was accepted by the World Health Organization (WHO) and is used to this day.

Historically, various measures were employed to control drinking habits, some of which were extreme. Examples include that of Liu Jun, a Chinese emperor who in 459 AD decreed that drinkers should be decapitated, and that of the caliph Hakim (996–1020 AD) who ordered all vines to be uprooted and stopped the import of alcohol into Egypt. Later attempts ranged from the promotion of abstinence to outright prohibition. The latter approach often backfired by driving production of distilled drinks underground and increasing criminal activity. By banning vodka in 1916, for example, Tsar Nicholas the Second of Russia may have precipitated his eventual demise, as the banning led to a disconsolate military.

The temperance movement of nineteenth-century England initially aimed to use moral persuasion rather than legislation to restrict the use of alcohol. Its history is a fascinating example of class struggle and conflict between extreme and moderate ideologies. Although initiated by the middle classes, seven working-class men under the leadership of Joseph Livesey (1794–1884), a social activist and philanthropist, advocated the more extreme position of teetotalism. These men, who took the pledge never to drink alcohol again, saw their movement as a way of advancing their status through upholding the Victorian ideals of self-control and self-denial. Many working class men also joined the 'Chartist' movement, which was a political movement seeking to win universal adult male suffrage. A large number of Chartists regarded teetotalism as an aid to obtaining political rights.

If the Chartist movement alienated many of the middle classes, the United Kingdom Alliance, which from 1853 lobbied for prohibition and the closure of public houses, was seen as a direct attack on the working class. However, unlike in the State of Maine in the USA, where the first prohibition law in the West was passed in 1851, the British Government overwhelmingly voted against a prohibition law in 1859. Despite this, the temperance movement continued to flourish in the UK, supported by prominent Victorian feminists concerned about the plight of women married to drunkards, by chapels and by people of all classes who recognised the social costs of liquor to their society. Apart from the human misery that excessive use of alcohol caused, it was also acknowledged that a growing industrialised society needed a workforce that was reliable and alert. Ironically, although the Church of England was certainly supportive of the temperance movement, it objected when the prohibitionists suggested that grape juice rather than wine should be used during services.

Attitudes and responses to alcoholism have been influenced by each epoch's prevailing view regarding causality. 'Inebriety', a term replaced by 'addiction' by the time of the First World War, was thought to be the result of degenerationism in the second half of the nineteenth century. 'Degeneration theory' postulated that acquired negative characteristics are not only passed on to the next generation but also accentuated in each subsequent generation, leading eventually to the extinction of the family. Such views contributed support to the eugenics movement and resulted in the obligatory sterilisation of alcoholics in Nazi Germany in the 1930s.

> **Discussion point**: In 1916, the newly-appointed president of the Society for the Study of Inebriation, Sir William Collins, described addiction as a 'disease of will'. What are current views about the causes of addiction and how much does the notion of personal choice figure in debates?

The influence of prevailing societal attitudes to alcohol is neatly shown by an examination of responses to women who drink. Recently, this has caused something of a moral panic, as can be inferred from a recent newspaper headline: 'Legacy of the ladette: now alarming rise in teenage promiscuity and abortions is linked with women's binge drinking' (S Borland, *Daily Mail*, 21 August 2010).

This sort of concern is not new. Irresponsible assertion of female personal choice has been a key concern of social commentators of the past such as William Hogarth in the eighteenth century, who highlighted the moral, social and health consequences of women's gin drinking in his famous cartoon *Gin Lane*. One newspaper in the 1740s alleged that over 84 000 children had died over the previous two decades because of gin drinking in women. The actual causes were more likely to have been poverty, infectious disease and polluted water, yet women were demonised for the supposed results of their drinking: promiscuity and the spread of syphilis, public disorder, non-submission to their husbands and the ill-health of their children.

The 'gin craze' first developed as a result of an act in 1690 for: Encourageing the Distilling of Brandy and Spirits from Come [which refers to any sort of grain] and for laying severall Dutyes on Low Wines or Spirits of the first Extraction, as war with France had rendered brandy temporarily unavailable. By 1713, any person could distil spirits without fear of prosecution. Gin selling was one of the few methods by which women could make a living in the cities, many of whom had moved from the country to urban environments hoping to improve their lot. Between 1720 and 1751, Parliament passed eight gin acts to both reduce consumption and to raise more tax to fund war activities. Unlicensed retailers were convicted as a result. Although most of these retailers were men, 80% of those convicted were women.

Why is this relevant?

- Legislation has often had unintended consequences.
- Arguments over how to control alcohol use are also those of political and societal ideologies. Finding the right balance between civil liberty and state control is a current challenge that was rehearsed in the discourses and legislation of Victorian England.
- It is difficult to understand issues concerning current usage of alcohol without knowledge of its cultural and historical background.
- Simplistically making one group in society a scapegoat for a particular issue is a feature of the past as well as now. This approach ignores underlying complex social and cultural parameters, which should be addressed first.

Further reading

Dillon P. *Gin: the much lamented death of Madame Geneva; the eighteenth century gin craze*. Boston, MA: Justin, Charles and Co; 2004.

Sournia JC. *A History of Alcoholism*. Hindley N, Stanton G, translators. Oxford: Basil Blackwell; 1990.

4

Friend or foe? Substance use

THE DEATH OF BILLIE CARLETON (1896–1918) IN NOVEMBER 1918 WAS the first big drug scandal of the twentieth century. The newspapers were full of details about her untimely death. This beautiful and frail young actress, who was well on her way to being a star at the age of 22, was found dead in her suite at the Savoy Hotel the night after attending the Victory Ball at the Royal Albert Hall. A court case heard that she had died of an overdose of cocaine that had been supplied by her dress designer and partner Reggie de Veulle and that she had been using cocaine and opium heavily for some time. Alcohol and drug misuse often coexist in today's society with either having the potential to lead to accidental death, as the following headline reminds us: 'Amy Winehouse found dead at her London flat aged 27' (BBC Newsbeat [website], 23 July 2011). Although this talented young woman died accidentally of alcohol intoxication, she regularly used heroin, cannabis and crack cocaine.

In the first decades of the twentieth century, cocaine sniffing and opium parties were fashionable in literary and theatrical circles, although a select committee on the use of cocaine concluded in 1917 that there was no evidence of serious use in the civilian or military population of Britain. This investigation had been prompted by a groundless anxiety that prostitutes were selling drugs to soldiers, leading to a cocaine 'epidemic'. By the 1920s, cocaine, rather than hashish or opium, was the fashionable drug. Carleton's death was a shock partly because it very publicly exposed the potential lethality of recreational drug use.

Mind-altering substances have been used throughout history. In the caves of Lascaux in southern France, Palaeolithic rock symbols and art may have been produced by shamans whose consciousness was altered by drugs or self-induced trance states. Some experts even suggest that the human ability to make symbols, which later led to the development of art and symbolic thinking, was facilitated by hallucinogenic drugs. There is clear evidence that the use of mind-altering drugs extends back to Ancient Greece and Rome, but this was chiefly for their medicinal benefits rather than hallucinogenic effects. Opium, which was originally grown in the Middle East, had spread to China and India by at least 800 AD. Cocaine came from South America and was a central feature of social and religious practices in the Inca Empire (1200–1553 AD). It spread to Europe together with tobacco and other vegetable species after the 'discovery' of the New

World in 1492. Coffee roasting was developed in about 1450 in Arabia, making it cheaper and more available to the West.

In time, cocaine, opium and coffee developed a significant commercial value and cultural cachet that trumped any later concerns about safety. This is well illustrated by the story of British opium smuggling to China. By the late eighteenth century, the East India Company had assumed control of all opium-growing areas of Bengal and Bihar in India and tried to popularise its use to increase company profits. British opium traders established depots in Chinese ports to import opium from India despite the country's emperor prohibiting its importation, consumption and sale. Illegal imports rose five-fold between 1821 and 1837, even though smokers and dealers could be executed; millions of Chinese became addicted and the economic decline of the country was blamed on this. The two wars directly related to the British opium trade that broke out in the ensuing decades were won by the British and resulted in China ceding Kowloon (Hong Kong) to Britain, opening their ports to foreign vessels and agreeing to the legalisation of opium in the Treaty of Tien-tsin in 1860.

Question 1: What is current Chinese government policy towards drug addicts?

In the West, opium, sometimes called 'laudanum', was a popular means of self-medication for medical conditions from the eighteenth century. Its medicinal uses had been well publicised in England by both William Buchan's *Domestic Medicine*, first published in 1769, and Dr John Jones' *The Mysteries of Opium Revealed* of 1770. Dover's Powder, which contained ipecacuanha and opium powder, was widely used for the next 150 years for colds and fevers. However, it was well known that users could become iatrogenically addicted; Samuel Johnson's wife, Tetty, became addicted, as did Mary Ann (née Todd) Lincoln, wife of Abraham Lincoln. Thomas De Quincy's book *Confessions of an English Opium-Eater*, which described in forensic detail his use of opium to relieve neuralgia, caused quite a stir on its publication in 1821, attracting both interest and condemnation. Concerns about drug use, particularly among the working class in the industrial cities, led to several public health inquiries between the 1820s and 1850s. One such heard how when an 'infant was 4 months old, she was so "wrankle" and thin that folk persuaded her [mother] to give it laudanum to bring it on' (Parssinnen TM, 1983).

The Pharmacy Act 1869 was passed to restrict sale of opiates to qualified pharmacists; by then, opium was cheaper than alcohol, partly because it attracted no tax on account of its medicinal status. At about the same time, the British Medical Association set up a committee to lobby for the compulsory detention of inebriates. In 1887, its supporters formed the Society for Study of Inebriety, which addressed addiction to both alcohol and drugs, through its publication, the *British Journal Of Inebriety* (which later became the *British Journal of Addiction*). The society promoted a disease model of addiction and recommended the need for treatment.

Question 2: What other explanatory models of addiction became popular in the second half of the nineteenth century?

Anti-opium sentiments in Britain continued to be fuelled by literary accounts such as Charles Dickens' first six episodes of *The Mysteries of Edwin Drood* (1870) and Oscar Wilde's *The Picture of Dorian Gray* (1891). The Anti-Opium League was organised against the 'evil' opium trade with China. The Shanghai Opium Commission of 1909, convened by the USA, addressed opium control in the Far East and led to the 1912 Hague Convention, which attempted to establish a worldwide system of narcotics control. This direction was later incorporated in the Treaty of Versailles after the First World War.

However, the medical profession's opinion of mind-altering drugs was not universally denigratory:

> Opium is used, rightly or wrongly, in many oriental countries, not as an idle or vicious indulgence but as a reasonable aid in the work of life. A patient of [mine] took [60 mg] of opium [every morning] . . . he persisted in this habit, as being one which gave him no conscious gratification or diversion, but *which toned and strengthened him for his deliberations and engagements* . . .
>
> A System of Medicine, Sir Thomas Clifford Allbutt, 1906
> emphasis in original.

Some physicians took the view that mind-altering drugs could be useful in developing the field of psychology. Silas Weir Mitchell (1829–1914), an American neurologist and writer, famous for his 'rest cure' for women with neurosis, wrote a paper describing the effects of a hallucinogenic plant which is now often referred to as mescal or peyote: 'The display which for an enchanted two hours followed was such that I find hopeless to describe in language which shall convey to others the beauty and splendour of what I saw' (Mitchell SW. Remarks on the Effects of Anhelonium lewenii (the 'mescal button'); *British Medical Journal*. 1896; **2**: 1626).

On reading Mitchell's account, the British social reformer, physician and psychologist Havelock Ellis (1859–1939) was prompted to try out mescal to see how it could expand perceptual experience. This interest was consonant with a growing curiosity about inner consciousness, which overlapped with the popular Victorian pursuit of esotericism, a means of understanding the hidden mysteries of the universe. Spiritual groups emerged, as modern off-shoots of Rosicrucianism, such as the Cabalist Order and the Hermetic Order of the Golden Dawn, which attracted literary figures such as the poet William Butler Yeats and authors like Arnold Bennett and Edith Nesbitt. These mystic groups were natural venues for recreational drug use.

Some physicians upheld the medical benefits of mind-altering drugs. For example, Thomas Clouston (1840–1915), a pioneer psychiatrist, won the Fothergillian Gold Medal in 1870 for his research on patients at the West Riding Pauper Lunatic Asylum that showed cannabis was therapeutically superior to opium. Walter Dixon, who researched the pharmacology of cannabis in the

1890s, took the view that 'hemp taken as an inhalation may be placed in the same category as coffee, tea or kola' (Dixon W. The pharmacology of Cannabis indica. *British Medical Journal*. 1899; **ii**: 1354–7). He was later a member of the Rolleston Committee on Morphine and Heroin, which was established to advise on the circumstances, if any, in which the supply of these drugs was medically advisable. By 1926, this committee's report came to the significant conclusion that addiction was 'a manifestation of disease and not a mere form of vicious indulgence'. Further, it endorsed a medical approach which advocated that most heroin and morphine addicts should be medically prescribed maintenance doses of opioids. The report commented that because so few criminal or lower class addicts existed, there was no need for criminal sanctioning and noted that most addicts were from the middle class or doctors (Paragraph 27, Departmental Committee on Morphine and Heroin Addiction (Rolleston) 1926).

Until the 1960s, the numbers of addicts remained low; only up to 1000 names per year were forwarded to the Home Office and most of these were medical personnel. The medical approach endorsed by the Rolleston committee became known as the 'British system' and was in stark contrast to the American penal approach. It worked because the problem was limited in size. However, with international drug dealing from the 1960s on, the numbers of heroin addicts rapidly rose.

Question 3: What were the consequences of the increase in heroin usage in the 1960s?

Why is this relevant?

- Attitudes towards drugs have varied enormously in the past, just as they do now. They are arguably shaped more by the cultural context than medical concerns.
- It is likely that people will always want to use mind-altering substances and no legislation will stop this completely.
- Today, some of us may be judgemental of the medical experimentation with drugs to expand and intensify human experience that occurred at the turn of the twentieth century; however, medical and societal curiosity about pharmaceutical methods to affect human performance and perception is ongoing. This is illustrated by the growing interest in developing cognitive enhancers, for example.

Further reading

Berridge V. Edwards G. *Opium and the People: opiate use and drug control policy in the nineteenth century and early twentieth century England*. London: Free Association Books; 1998.

Ghosh A. *River of Smoke* [novel]. London: John Murray; 2011.

Hodgson B. *In the Arms of Morpheus: the tragic history of laudanum, morphine and patent medicines*. New York, NY: Firefly; 2001.

Parssinnen TM. *Secret Passions, Secret Remedies: narcotic drugs in British society 1820–1930*. Philadelphia: Institute for the Study of Human Issues; Manchester: Manchester University Press; 1983. p. 44.

5

Before vitamins: the elusive ingredient

WHILE PRECISE KNOWLEDGE OF VITAMINS WAS DENIED TO PEOPLE before the early twentieth century, the medical problems induced by dietary deficiencies were plain for all to see, and remedial actions were recognised and implemented. For example, in Ancient Egypt, liver was eaten to cure night blindness. The most obvious complaint in Britain and Europe occurred among populations with limited access to fresh fruit and vegetables. With hindsight, the most vulnerable group comprised the soldiers and sailors of the British Royal and Merchant navies as well as those of private fleets who spent months at a time on board ships subjected to a restricted diet of preserved or long-lasting foodstuffs. Under such conditions, scurvy presented after as little as 6 weeks and had a drastic impact on men's bodily capabilities.

In early eighteenth-century Britain, there was a range of ideas about the causes of scurvy. Damp and cold air, noxious gas, inactivity or exhaustion were all regarded as dangerous, but the potential risks of an inadequate diet were also considered, and, eventually, experiments were undertaken with different types of supplements. Sauerkraut and malt infusions were tried and typically found wanting, but the 'small' (low alcohol) beer that was the main form of liquid intake on board ships also had an antiscorbutic effect. A process of trial and error eventually identified fresh vegetables as preventative and acidic fruits, particularly the juice of lemons, as effective in treating scurvy.

It was difficult for contemporaries to theorise *why* fruit and vegetables had antiscorbutic properties. The perceptive doctor Thomas Trotter (1760–1832) wrote in 1797 that 'vegetable matter imparts a *something* to the body' [emphasis in the original] and so postulated the presence of the substance that would later be labelled 'vitamin C'. Unfortunately, without a convincing explanation for the power of this unnamed 'something', the rationale for costly improvements to shipboard diets was unproven and unpopular with navy quartermasters. In the 1790s, lemon juice became the most important substance for both treating and preventing scurvy, because it was easier to transport and keep than a supply of vegetables for a lengthy sea journey. Naval doctors became convinced by the antiscorbutic results of using lemon and citrus juices, but ensuring a constant supply of juice for the whole navy was a logistical nightmare at first. However, it became a matter of national identification when British sailors acquired the nickname 'limeys'.

> **Question**: Why might the improving health of the British navy and marine forces in the late eighteenth century have made a dramatic difference to the nation?

Other forms of dietary deficiency, particularly vitamin B deficiencies such as beriberi, were unlikely to present in the British population at any time prior to 1950 owing to the wheat-based staples that formed the diet of most ordinary working people. Bread was the main source of carbohydrate for the majority well into the twentieth century, while potatoes (and fried potato chips) did not even become a familiar dietary component outside of Ireland until the later nineteenth century. This is in marked contrast to East Asia, where beriberi was and remains a real problem among the poor, because the dietary staple remains white rice (*see* Chapter 6 in this section, 'Green sickness and other anaemias').

Why is this relevant?

- Knowledge of vitamins is a relatively recent addition to human understandings of diet.
- Traditional eating patterns can be difficult to alter, particularly if any undue cost is involved and even when health benefits can be proven.
- Widespread modern knowledge about the best-publicised vitamins and application of this knowledge (e.g. the recommendation to eat at least five portions of fruit and vegetables per day) may conceal much poorer appreciation of other substances such as vitamin K.
- In contrast, the pharmaceutical industry has persuaded the public of the health benefits of supplementary vitamins, making exaggerated claims regarding their protective value, such as for heart disease or cancers, many of which have been proven unfounded.

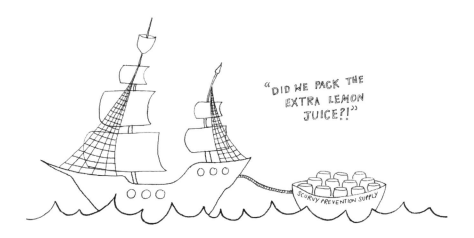

The pleasures of life: food, drink, drugs and sex

Further reading

Trotter T. *Medicinia Nautica. An essay on the disease of seamen.* London: T. Cadell and W. Davies; 1797.

Vale B, Edwards G. *Physician to the Fleet: the life and times of Thomas Trotter 1760–1832.* Woodbridge: Boydell Press; 2011.

6

Green sickness and other anaemias

Her vestal livery is but sick and green

Shakespeare, *Romeo and Juliet*, Act 2, Scene 2, line 8

THIS DESCRIPTION OF JULIET IS A REFERENCE TO 'GREEN SICKNESS', A common affliction of the sixteenth century, which was regarded by many in the first part of the century to be a digestive disorder. This changed when Johannes Lange (1485–1565), a well-known German physician, wrote a letter of advice in 1554 to the father of a sickly daughter in which he described it as a 'disease of virgins' characterised primarily by lack of menstruation, a greenish pallor, weakness and anorexia. He cited a newly translated text by Hippocrates (c. 460–c. 370 BC), 'On the diseases of virgins', as his authority. In fact, Hippocrates did not describe the same symptoms as Lange but did advise that the health problems of pubescent girls were best treated by bloodletting and marriage. Within the humoral theory of disease, this was logical given the belief that suppressed menstrual flow caused rotting and toxic vapours; it was thought that bloodletting got rid of accumulated menstrual blood and that marriage promoted normal menstrual flow (*see* Section 3, Chapter 1, 'On "the blob" and other menstrual euphemisms'). Although there were some dissenters from this view – such as Thomas Sydenham (1624–89), who in 1681 classified it as a hysterical disease, for which he advocated iron – green sickness continued to be thought of as a disorder of pubescence. In the *Dictionary of the Vulgar Tongue* of 1811 it is defined as 'a disease of maids occasioned by celibacy'. Professor Jean Verandal of Montpellier introduced the term 'chlorosis' (derived from the Greek *chloros*, meaning 'green') in 1615 but 'green sickness' remained the popular term.

By the mid-nineteenth century, views were changing. In 1872, Sir Andrew Clark of The London Hospital concluded that sudden growth and menarche accounted for the disease. Then, in 1895, a pathologist, Ralph Stockman, showed that iron contributed to the synthesis of haemoglobin and suggested that menstrual loss together with a poor diet caused green sickness. Some 40 years later, Arthur J Patek and Clark W Heath demonstrated that chlorosis was hypochromic

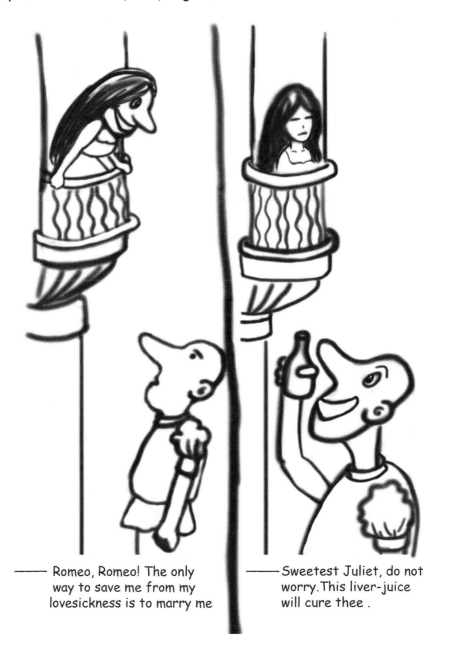

anaemia; however, although iron was often an effective treatment, some physicians were not entirely persuaded by a purely physiological explanation for all cases. A variation was proposed towards the end of the nineteenth century – chloro-anorexia – which was thought to be psychogenic in origin. Of course, today we might re-diagnose chloro-anorexia as anorexia nervosa, given that patients share the symptoms originally described by Lange; in such a case, anaemia would be a secondary physical consequence of anorexia nervosa.

Discussion point: It has been argued that a disease of virgins, which responded to marriage, was a convenient way of handling sexuality of young women at a time when early marriage was socially desirable. Could other 'diseases' of the past or present be seen as useful social constructs?

A report of sickle-cell anaemia in a Ghanaian family dated 1670 exists in the literature. The condition was well known to the African people, particularly in Nigeria where sufferers were called *ogbanje* – 'children who come and go'. It was believed that *ogbanje* could reincarnate. The malevolent *ogbanje* were the ones who in the past realised that they could not succeed in the world and so decided to die in order to return to heaven but found entry was denied them. So they formed a spirit society, living in the baobab trees, and sometimes decided to be reborn and live with a human family. Before doing so, they had to pledge to the other *ogbanje* that they would return on a certain date; this date was usually one of particular significance to the family into which they were reborn, thereby causing maximum grief. Most afflicted children died before the age of 5 years. Families who were used to losing their children tended to give names that reflected their apprehension such as Malomo ('do not die again') or Kokumo ('he will not die again'). Once dead, a witch doctor mutilated the child so that his kindred spirits would reject the child and he or she would, on rebirth, live out his or her life in the physical world (*see* Section 5, Chapter 2, 'Two steps forward, one step back: disability'). Even today, this culturally defined phenomenon remains, resulting in some mothers denying their infants medical care. There still seems to be some cultural resistance to the idea that (in many cases) their children are suffering from sickle-cell anaemia. This is illustrated in the response to a query on a Nigerian online forum from a young man who has fallen in love with a girl who has told him she is *ogbanje*:

> ogbanje ogbanje!!!!!!1 hmmm this one na serious matta oo
>
> [...]
>
> In some quarters, they are simply called abiku, others generalise them as witches and many other names depending on the area.
>
> now the most important thing here is to prove if this lady is really ogbanje
>
> ...
>
> my take is this,
> 1. [s]he has right to life, not just live, becos she ws created by and for God and not the devil, she simply needs deliverance, prayers and assistance(care, love(agape), friendlinesss and teaching-general things and the word of God]. she needs real help
> 2. poster shd thnak God he already knows this b4 going into the relationship, otherwise a lot of things may be hppening in his/their llife that he may not understand or comprehend. so he is already forewarned.
> 3. but now the main isssue is that she is not ready to come out of the cult,
> 4. poster shd discuss with his pastor becos na serious matter

my sincere prayer is for the lady to agree to come out and be free cos she is
under reall bondage, although she may not agree to this now until she is fully
delivered. its a whole lot of issues and the matter na be small one,

I will get back with more info and by Gods grace all will end well,

goldboy, 'Re: I'm in love with an ogbanje' [online post],
Nairaland Forum [website], 18 January 2008

In 1904, a young first-year dental student from Grenada, Walter Clement
Noel, was admitted to hospital with anaemia. He came under the care of
Professor James Herrick (1861–1954), whose junior doctor, Ernest Edward
Irons (1877–1959), observed 'peculiar elongated and sickle-shaped cells' in his
blood (Kelly FB. 1959). Although re-admitted several times, Noel completed his
studies and practised until his death in 1916 of pneumonia. In 1927, E Vernon
Hahn and Elizabeth Gillespie discovered that red blood cells from persons with
the disease could be made to sickle by removing oxygen. It was also noted that
although relatives of the patient often had this trait of sickling when deprived
of oxygen, they had no disease. This condition became known as 'sickle trait'.
The hereditary nature of the disease was not confirmed until 1949. Its association with haemoglobin was discovered in 1951 by Linus Pauling (1901–94) and
Harvey Hano, who observed that the structure of haemoglobin, the protein that
carried oxygen, was different in people with sickle-cell disorder. Vernon Ingram
(1924–2006) then identified the substituted amino acid in 1956.

Question: What made the pathology of sickle-cell anaemia particularly novel?

In the 1850s, Thomas Addison (1793–1860) described a lethal form of anaemia
related to a pathological gastric mucosa associated with the absence of acid in the
stomach – today this would be referred to as 'pernicious anaemia'. The signs were
a macrocytic anaemia, glossitis and neurological symptoms such as paraesthesia
and an odd gait. Interest was stimulated and several papers were published in
the latter half of the nineteenth century, which described the clinical picture in
much the same way as we would today. The aetiology was debated but Samuel
Fenwick (1821–1902) came closest to speculating correctly in his book of 1880,
On Atrophy of the Stomach and on The Nervous Affections of the Digestive Organs,
that it was not atrophy per se but the loss of a secretion from gastric juice that led
to the disease. In the early 1920s, George Whipple's (1878–1976) research using
experimental animals demonstrated that the most effective dietary addition for
chronic anaemia was raw liver. In 1926, George Minot (1885–1950) and William
P Murphy (1892–1987) reported that 45 patients were cured by this diet. They
had taken careful dietary histories from their patients and discovered that meat
had been excluded from their normal diet. All three received the Nobel Prize in
1934. In 1928, Edwin Joseph Cohn (1892–1953) prepared a concentrated liver
extract, which made treatment less onerous than having to eat large quantities
of raw liver and drink liver juice.

In 1936, William Castle (1867–1962) at Harvard revisited Fenwick's idea of a key substance deficiency, postulating an 'intrinsic factor' in the gastric mucosa that was necessary for the normal absorption of an 'extrinsic factor' in the liver. In a rather indelicate experiment, he ate raw hamburger each morning, which he then regurgitated an hour later. This he then fed to patients with vitamin B_{12} deficiency. Those who were given non-regurgitated raw hamburger failed to improve. On publishing a series of papers based on 61 cases, he announced that:

> If beef muscle and gastric juice are administered without opportunity for contact, they are not effective. It is obvious, therefore, that the activity of mixtures of beef muscle and gastric juice cannot be due to the simple addition of two sub threshold substances but requires an interaction between them.

In 1948, Castle isolated B_{12} (cobalamin), his extrinsic factor. Dorothy Hodgkin (1910–94) described vitamin B_{12}'s molecular structure in 1956, for which she received the Nobel Prize. Successful chemical synthesis was achieved in 1971. The elusive 'intrinsic factor's' structure was identified in the 1970s and found to be a glycoprotein secreted by the parietal cells of the stomach.

Why is this relevant?

- The story of green sickness demonstrates how hard it can be to differentiate cause and effect, particularly when there are different pathological conditions with similar presentations.
- The social construct of green sickness advocated a 'treatment' – namely, early marriage – which suited the cultural, and possibly economic, demands of the time. Critics of medical practice today often complain that normal physical states are conveniently defined as illnesses to satisfy prevailing social needs. The pharmaceutical industry is then accused of encouraging this by introducing medication for spurious disease entities.
- The sickle-cell story demonstrates how constructs of illness can be widely different across cultures. The challenge in finding a constructive dialogue between them continues.

Further reading

Kelly FB. Ernest Edward Irons, 1877–1959. *Proc. Inst. Med Chic.* 1959; **22**: 326–328.

King H. *The Disease of Virgins: green sickness, chlorosis and the problems of puberty.* London and New York, NY: Routledge; 2004.

7

The 'single body' and changing understandings of sexuality

THE HUMAN BODY MAY NOT HAVE CHANGED AT ALL IN EVOLUTIONARY terms throughout the whole of recorded history, but the way that people have understood bodies has undergone important shifts. In the twenty-first century, anatomical study and microscopy mean that male and female bodies are recognised as containing different structures that have distinct reproductive functions. In the seventeenth century, people saw their bodies in other ways; most importantly, they thought male and female bodies were essentially the same.

Bodies were thought to be governed by four humours (*see* Section 6, Chapter 1, 'Early Greek and Roman contributions') and men and women were considered to enjoy different balances of those humours. Women were thought to be composed of cold and wet humours, while hot and dry humours were uppermost in men's bodies, with each individual comprised of a different specific composition. However, the human frames that contained these humours were regarded as identical. The male penis and testes could exist on the outside of the hot male body but were retained within the colder female as the birth canal and the ovaries. In this way, men's and women's bodies were construed as mirror images of the same material.

This comprehension of the human body had important implications for sexuality. Sexual desire was held to be strongest in women on the presumption that cold and leaky bodies would always seek to acquire more of the hot dry properties of semen. In this way, sex could be understood as strengthening for women but as a process that weakened men. These ideas fuelled the notions that masturbation was exceedingly dangerous for men and that women might suffer grievously from insufficient sexual activity. Thus, sexual health was regarded as vital for bodily health, and beneficial 'balance' in this context entailed measured engagement of adults in sex within the institution of marriage.

Historian Thomas Laqueur has argued that the single-body model had been replaced by a two-body understanding by about 1820. However, this did not come about as a consequence of medical progress but instead from a societal need to see women as decisively different to men. Others have modified his conclusions, arguing that change did not occur suddenly towards the end of the eighteenth century but rather took place gradually as humoral understandings of the body declined. In either case, ideas about women's sexuality underwent a complete revolution so that 'normal' women were seen as sexually passive by the end of the nineteenth century.

> **Question**: Using Internet dictionaries of English phrases, research current thoughts about the origin of the saying 'lie back and think of England'. What is the most popular explanation of this expression epitomising female passivity? Which one do you think is right?

Heterosexual activity has never been the sole expression of sexuality, but it would be anachronistic to describe people as 'gay' before the twentieth century. Understandings of sexual identity, or the role of sexual activity in forming identity, have also undergone profound changes. Sodomy was a felony punishable by the death penalty in the seventeenth century and beyond, so the single-body model was no source of solace to men who were attracted to men – but then, 'sodomy' was a catch-all phrase that might encompass widely differing practices (perhaps including fellatio). It was also very difficult to prove in English law, since it required two witnesses and both partners were liable for prosecution (so neither was encouraged to report the other), which meant that the risk of being prosecuted for consensual intercourse of any kind between adults was slim. It is probable that there was a significant disparity between the severity of the law and lay tolerance of a range of practices. This was particularly likely when sequestered populations could not choose from among a range of potential sexual partners (for example, populations on board ships who did not set foot on land for months at a time).

However, Tim Hitchcock has argued that the two-body model encouraged a narrowing phallocentric definition of what was permissible between consenting adults and that this definition became increasingly entrenched in popular culture. Sex for the purposes of reproduction between a man and a woman became considered normal and over-wrote older patterns of non-penetrative sex that might be involved in either 'vigorous courtship' or casual encounters, such as mutual masturbation with opposite- or same-sex partners. By 1800, the acceptable variety of sexual activity had become closely proscribed, with negative consequences for both men and women who deviated from this.

Why is this relevant?
- Some of the assumptions about sexual 'normality' that dominated the twentieth century were not based on traditional common-sense ideas of longstanding but were themselves eighteenth- or nineteenth-century constructions.
- Sexual activity between same-sex partners was denigrated under both bodily models, but the two-body model made life more difficult for men attracted to men or women attracted to women, since it encouraged the notion that the only legitimate sexual activity was the penile penetration of a vagina.

Further reading

Hitchcock T. *English Sexualities, 1700–1800.* Basingstoke: Macmillan; 1997.

Laqueur T. *Making Sex: body and gender from the Greeks to Freud.* Cambridge, MA: Harvard University Press; 1990.

Section 3

The facts of life: women health and medicine

1

'On the blob' and other menstrual euphemisms

MENSTRUATION IS A COMPONENT OF FEMALE IDENTITY AND SEXUAL health, so it exerts a significant influence over the life experiences of adolescent girls and adult women. It is a biological process which has gone largely unchanged across human history, although the age at which periods begin or end is determined in part by nutrition and lifestyle and the intervals between periods were probably lengthened for women suffering nutritional deprivation.

Belief systems imbue menstruation with different meanings. A typical position adopted by more than one world faith is that menstrual blood is unclean and/or that women who are bleeding cannot obtain or sustain a state of grace. Historically, the biological fact of menstruation has supported perceptions of women as inferior to men. In this context, women have found a variety of ways to allude to the onset, process and cessation of periods that, unsurprisingly, tend to use allusive and evasive language rather than direct and clear labelling.

These euphemisms are not solely a product of modern life. In seventeenth-century England, menstruation could be referred to as 'the flowers' (a picturesque reference to the blooming of red on the thighs or an optimistic assumption that 'fruit', in the form of a child, would follow), 'the courses' (a regular event) or the 'monthly infirmity' (in other words, a form of malady). In the privacy of

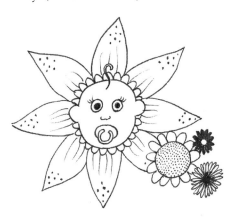

documents such as diaries, both men and women alluded simply to 'them'. The world's only Museum of Menstruation and Women's Health in New York has an online forum for gathering words and phrases meaning menstruation. Examples include 'coming on', 'a visit from aunt Flo' and 'on the rag'. In some parts of the world, the association of the colour red with communism gives rise to phrases implying that Communist Party representatives have arrived!

Question: What terms have you heard in use to refer to menstruation? Is this a question that you could ask your mother, grandmother or other female relations without embarrassment in the interests of historical research?

There is also a long history of medical commentary on and concern about the absence of menstruation. When periods did not begin when anticipated, young unmarried women might be diagnosed with 'green sickness'. When periods stopped but the cause was not an evident pregnancy, an array of measures could be used to restore them, including a prescription for sexual activity. In all eras, restoration of menstruation has been regarded as vital for women's physical and mental health.

Why is this relevant?

- Relatively open discussion of menstrual health and sanitary goods has only been a feature of social life in Britain since around 1990, and in many cultures and communities it remains taboo.
- Practitioners need to be aware of the variety of ways patients might allude to menstruation.
- Amenorrhoea can give rise to diverse assumptions and responses among patients according to the meanings they ascribe to it.

Further reading

Crawford P. Attitudes to menstruation in seventeenth-century England. *Past and Present*. 1981; **91**: 47–73.
www.mum.org

2

How not to have a baby: the history of contraception

CONTRACEPTION HAS A FRAUGHT HISTORY, OWING TO THE MYSTERIES surrounding the mechanisms of conception and the general taboos covering discussion of sexual activity. Few writers leave direct evidence of their methods for inhibiting conception, even in their most private diaries or correspondence. These forms of reticence are compounded by the influence exerted by different faiths over the course of history; for example, even delays to marriage were criticised by the pious of both Catholic and Protestant faiths (if for rather different reasons). Contraception might be alluded to remotely but as a comparable sin to infanticide.

Therefore, the history of contraceptive activities, while ancient, is largely hidden. Some methods have undoubtedly been used throughout human history, including coitus interruptus, abstention, douching or pessaries, plus inducement of abortion in the early weeks of pregnancy. The manner and spread of these techniques is uncertain, and their efficacy was highly unreliable. Historian Hera Cook argues that contraceptive activity shifted from communal or indirect control by communities to more direct and effective control by individuals. This means that for most of history people have relied on postponement of sexual activity (policed via marriage), pervasive cultures of breastfeeding (inhibiting ovulation) and tacit acceptance of prostitution as mechanisms of general population control. Individuals may have sought prophylactic or abortifacient strategies, such as consumption of the herb pennyroyal, but these did not make a significant difference to populations overall. However, from the nineteenth century, devices such as condoms, sponges and douches were understood more widely and used more regularly, and these eventually had a discernible impact on the birth rate in Western countries.

Question: Condoms made from cloth and other substances like sheep gut were reportedly used before 1800 but not for contraceptive purposes: what were their wearers using them for?

In 1832, a physician from New England called Charles Knowlton published

Fruits of Philosophy, or the Private Companion of Young Married People. Despite its very vague title, this book was in fact the first survey of contraceptive techniques published since approximately the second century AD. It was an exceedingly popular publication and quickly crossed the Atlantic; a pirated version was available in England from about 1833. It was read fairly widely, by working people as well as by the prosperous, but it is not clear that its recommendations were adopted. Knowlton advocated using a douche containing a basic form of spermicide that may well have been effective, but unfortunately it was also a complicated solution to make for ordinary people living in crowded accommodation on a tight budget.

The first birth-control organisation in the world, the Malthusian League, was founded in Britain in 1877. It explicitly promoted the use of contraception within marriage but appealed more to the middle classes and tended to alienate members of the labour movement.

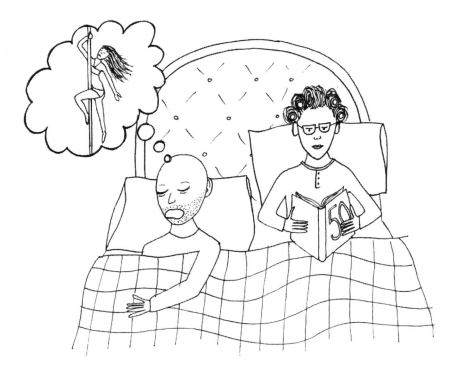

Doctors were largely opposed to the spread of contraceptive knowledge on the grounds that it tended to deprive them of both scientific authority and potential patients. Dr Henry Allbutt was even removed from the medical register after he published *The Wife's Handbook* in 1885; the book featured condoms, douches, sponges and early diaphragms. From the 1880s, the manufacture of vulcanised rubber on an industrial scale meant that condoms and diaphragms became more readily available and more efficient but opinion among medical practitioners remained trenchant. In 1901, the *British Medical Journal* condemned all forms of contraception as unnatural, injurious and degrading (The French and English birth-rates. *British Medical Journal* 29 June 1901: 1629). It fell to Marie Stopes, a botanist and later sexologist, to disseminate birth-control information more widely in Britain from the 1920s.

Why is this relevant?

- Birth control has been complicated historically by both general reticence on sexual matters and the concerns of specific social and religious groups.
- In the past and the present, some sections of the public have conflated the availability of contraception with permission to act promiscuously.
- The innovation of the female contraceptive pill in the 1960s was merely the next development in a long history of contraceptive technology to enable individuals to manage conception.

Further reading

Cook H. *The Long Sexual Revolution: English women, sex and contraception 1800–1975*. Oxford: Oxford University Press; 2004.
McLaren A. *Birth Control in Nineteenth-Century England*. London: Croom Helm; 1978.

3

'The sperm of men is full of small children' and other early ideas about conception

SEXUAL INTERCOURSE HAS BEEN UNDERSTOOD AS A PRECURSOR TO human reproduction for thousands of years but the specific cellular processes at work have only recently been appreciated. Before the development of advanced microscopy, people were forced to imagine what might take place and their imagination ran riot in some cases.

By the late seventeenth century, anatomical study of ovaries, fallopian tubes and testes via dissection ensured that there was a basic perception of human 'seed', but there was disagreement about the respective roles of ova and sperm. Historian Lisa Forman-Cody has described the most prominent theories about conception, which were debated in Britain by, among others, members of the Royal Society of London. The traditional explanation expounded by Galen (129–c. 200 AD), Aristotle (384–322 BC) and many of their contemporaries was that the two seeds met in the womb and operated in concert to generate human life. This idea gave equal significance to both male and female participants, but commentators diverged on the details: some thought that recognisable organs developed sequentially, while others held that all features of the new organism were generated simultaneously (to create a miniature but perfect human). The other, newer and (with hindsight) less accurate notion was that the whole future individual was suspended and enveloped by either the ova or a sperm. This view therefore saw conception as a spur to growth only rather than a developmental process.

Some pioneers in the field made impressive intuitive leaps in the absence of hard evidence. Antony van Leeuwenhoek (1632–1723), a Dutch businessman and author, published the first drawings of human sperm as a result of microscopic observation and, ironically, was mistakenly credited with the view in the title to this chapter – that sperm contained small children; however, he argued correctly that sperm was responsible for determining the sex of the new individual.

> **Question**: Why might people have been worried on theological grounds by the idea that every sperm contained a preformed human?

Whatever the initial processes of conception, there was widespread agreement in the seventeenth and eighteenth centuries that events during pregnancy, especially shocks or surprises to expectant mothers, could have a negative effect on infants. Women were encouraged to foster calm placid thoughts and were urged to avoid imagining or dwelling on distress. If a pregnant mother witnessed something shocking, ugly, violent or upsetting, it was thought that her child might be born 'monstrous' (the term then used for 'physical malformation').

Why is this relevant?

- The reproduction process is still surrounded by mystery and uncertainty. In the twenty-first century, the human genome has been mapped and medicine can provide sophisticated fertility treatment, yet the conception of children is never guaranteed.
- Notions about the emotional relationship of an embryo during gestation to the outside world remain, hence the suggestion to expectant mothers that they talk to their babies or play them music.
- Modern medical testing *may* reveal foetal congenital disabilities, but not all conditions can be detected by testing.

Further reading

Cody LF. *Birthing the Nation: sex, science and the conception of eighteenth-century Britons*. Oxford: Oxford University Press; 2007.

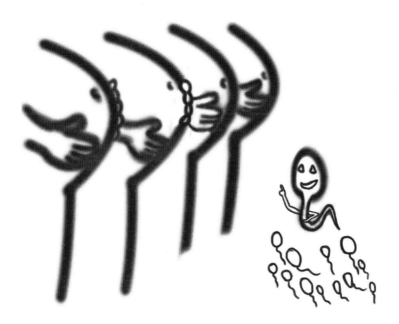

_____Fellows, we should be proud of what we have achieved!

4

Labour: temporary pain but permanent debility?

CHILDBIRTH HURTS – A LOT. THE DILATION OF THE OPENING AT THE base of the uterus and the passage of one or more infants along the birth canal, in addition to the muscular contractions required to facilitate birth, occasions pain unlike any other. Even women who have suffered wounds, surgery or disablement are unlikely to have suffered anything quite like it. The experience of this form of pain may *potentially* be subject to difference across the centuries, if women in the past understood their pain differently (in a context in which no anaesthesia was available), but this would be difficult to prove and generally seems improbable, especially since seventeenth- and eighteenth-century sources describe labour as the time of women's 'crying out'.

In 1915, the British Women's Co-operative Guild published a unique book entitled *Maternity: letters from working women*, a compilation of 160 letters from ordinary working-class women detailing their experiences of maternity from first conception through to the end of their reproductive lives. The letters provide poignant testimony to the fact that, in the generation before the First World War, sexual knowledge was difficult to come by, and variably distributed among the population. A number of women reflected on the information that might have been forthcoming from their own mothers but was not, owing to maternal absence or cultural reticence about reproductive health.

The pains of labour are referenced in this collection, but the aftermath of birth is given much more prominence as a source of longstanding suffering. Some women wrote about multiple unfettered conceptions, while others focused on the trials of bringing up a large family on a small wage. A set of letters speak movingly about the long-term physical tolls levied by single or repeated pregnancies, exacerbated by a lack of basic medical awareness. One woman wrote:

> I had no mother to talk to me, or for me to ask questions, . . . after the birth of my second child, I was a cripple for nearly twelve months . . . now I can call it mock modesty on my part . . . (72)

Another was more explicit:

> But after the birth of my first baby I suffered from falling womb, and the torture of that was especially cruel when at closet, in more than I can describe; and quite by accident I learnt that other mothers I met were not suffering the same. My baby was ten months old when I told the doctor, who said I ought to have told him before, and he soon put me right (38)

Thus, this correspondent's assumptions about a woman's lot in life meant that she suffered in silence for months. When she sought medical advice, the doctor even contrived to imply that her sufferings were her own fault. But lessons about openness in matters of sexual health were hard won if they were won at all. Even having been asked direct questions about postnatal health, the woman prefaced her account with the anxious comment, 'I hope this communication will not offend in any way'.

> **Question**: How common is it for women to suffer some degree of pelvic-organ prolapse? What are the other symptoms in addition to pain when going to the toilet, as was described in 1915?

The letters were sent in response to a questionnaire issued to members or former members of the Co-operative Women's Guild to provide evidence to support a scheme for maternal and infant welfare. An outline scheme devised by the Local Government Board in 1914 covered the need for antenatal clinics, home visiting, maternity hospitals and postnatal treatment. While the advice was not heeded everywhere, many towns began to make provision for mothers and infants.

Why is this relevant?

- Maternal health remains a concern for the international community, particularly since maternal mortality remains a potent indicator of national well-being (or otherwise).
- After delivery, mothers may feel that the medical focus has shifted away from her body to that of her baby. While a measure of this is inevitable, maternal health remains essential for the welfare of the baby, so women must be given every opportunity to regain and maintain physical well-being after birth.
- Maternity welfare and health provision form a costly component of state welfare systems, and while the principle is rarely challenged, the forms of delivery can vary dramatically in practice.

Further reading

Davies ML, editor. *Maternity: letters from working women.* London: Virago Press; 1989.

Fashion and forceps? The medicalisation of childbirth

IN 1650, BABIES WERE ALWAYS DELIVERED BY FEMALE MIDWIVES WHO fulfilled a social function as much as a medical one. Male doctors were only called in to attend births when the life of either the mother or the baby had been despaired, and the other life required drastic intervention to be saved. By 1800, though, the majority of prosperous families employed a male medical practitioner to deliver expectant mothers. How did this shift occur? Adrian Wilson has pointed to the impact of both fashion and forceps to explain changing attitudes.

Forceps were first invented by Peter Chamberlen (1560–1631) in Paris in the first half of the seventeenth century, but he did not advertise their design or usage. Instead, they were a well-kept secret and only used by Chamberlen or his apprentices. The Chamberlen family moved to London and eventually a publication of 1733 contained illustrations of his invention and an explanation of their function (Chapman E. *An Essay on the Improvement of Midwifery*. London: 1733). They comprised two long unhinged-but-interlocking pieces of curved metal, which could be inserted into the birth canal then used to grasp and exert traction on an infant. In this way, forceps allowed trained male practitioners to tackle difficult foetal presentations and to achieve positive outcomes for both mothers and infants (rather than their presiding over tragic childbirth events).

But male doctors were expensive. They tended to charge 10 shillings and six-pence, or a 'guinea' (one pound and one shilling, in pre-decimal coinage), whereas female midwives typically charged between two and five shillings to attend a delivery. Ironically, these differential charges did not secure the female midwife's position. Instead, eighteenth-century society came to regard male practitioners as properly (reassuringly) expensive and female midwives as charging a lower fee for a lower-grade service. In this way, it became a statement of conspicuous consumption, or 'fashionable', to employ a man at the onset of labour.

Question: Forceps are still unhinged but interlocking. Why?

Female practitioners regarded the encroachment of men on their occupational territory with dismay. Some women went into print to deprecate the use of forceps and other obstetrical instruments. Elizabeth Nihell (1723–?), for example, argued that childbirth should not be mechanical and emphasised the softness of women's hands for the task (Nihell E. *A Treatise on the Art of Midwifery.* 1760). Other critics of man-midwives reproached the over-eager use of instruments and even insinuated that male practitioners regarded deliveries as an opportunity to start seducing other men's wives! None of these charges made any difference; men still became the preferred choice for deliveries among prosperous families.

Why is this relevant?

● The changing status of childbirth, from a sociable, female event to a medical masculine one, took place via a combination of doctors' uses of new techniques *and* patients selecting the practitioner they perceived to be the best for the task. *However*, this does not rule out the possibility that both impulses were informed by underlying misogyny (expressed by doctors and the husbands of parturient mothers), and sexism of this sort certainly continues into the twenty-first century.

Further reading

Donnison J. *Midwives and Medical Men: a history of inter-professional rivalries and women's rights.* New York, NY: Schoken; 1977.

Wilson A. *The Making of Man-Midwifery: childbirth in England, 1660–1770.* Cambridge, MA: Harvard University Press; 1995.

6

How midwives became 'gamps'

IN 1802, THE REPUTATIONS OF MIDWIVES WERE NOT VERY HIGH IN medical and socially elite circles, but they were still well-regarded among ordinary working- and middle-class people. By 1902, midwives were collectively known by the derogatory label 'gamps' and that year became subject to legislative control for the first time. The new legislation was a mixed blessing for midwives, since it conferred professional registration on trained women but placed a substantial minority of (potentially hostile) medical men on the new Central Midwives Board. How did this happen?

The low opinion that doctors held of midwives in the early nineteenth century was dictated in part by competition: male practitioners, or 'accoucheurs', strived to secure lucrative deliveries among wealthy patients and replace female practitioners. This encouraged a low-level war of words between male and female midwives. But then in 1843, Charles Dickens published *The Life and Adventures of Martin Chuzzlewit* and gave the world Sarah Gamp. This character was a midwife, monthly nurse and occasional night nurse among the poor and lower-middle-class people and was invested with all of the negative attributes sometimes associated with such women. Her appearance was grotesque and her dress was chaotic, but her moral failings were the most striking aspect of the character for readers. She was portrayed putting her own needs above those of her patients, being a callous and semi-violent 'carer' and constantly in a state of insobriety. Unfortunately for female midwives, the word 'gamp' entered the English language and became a byword for slovenly, ignorant, unhygienic and immoral behaviour by nurses and midwives, particularly the latter.

The image of Sarah Gamp was seized by male practitioners and mobilised to drive down the reputation of the female midwife, and this was almost certainly unjust in relation to most of the women who were denigrated. It was undoubtedly the case, however, that lots of female midwives could not read or write; it is by no means certain that this rendered them unfit to practise in the late nineteenth-century context.

> **Question**: From your own training and practice, have you encountered present-day tensions between midwives and obstetricians? How does any conflict between the two practitioners manifest?

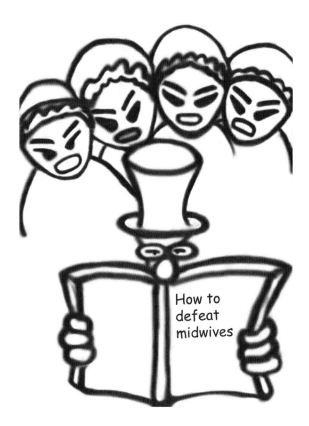

The Midwives Act 1902 was the product of a bitter struggle between a vocal subset of male practitioners who sought to remove women entirely from the task of infant delivery, and a group of socially elite individuals (supported by a handful of embattled male practitioners) who were determined to see women's employment rights and career prospects recognised. In the 12 years preceding the act, *The Lancet*, the *British Medical Journal* and other influential medical publications were vociferous in their opposition to recognition for midwives and were determined that if midwifery registration were to occur, it should be wholly governed by the General Medical Council. Multiple parliamentary Bills were introduced and thrown out, until, in 1902, public opinion began to form decisively behind the pro-registration group and members of parliament evinced both sympathy for the latest bill and considerable irritation with the medical profession. The resulting act was hailed a success by women's movements, but burdened midwives with requirements for unceasing professional *and personal* probity.

Why is this relevant?

- The 2001 census showed that only 1% of qualified midwives in Britain were male: the historic gender divide remains.
- Pervasive anecdotal evidence supports the idea that there can still be a good deal of conflict between obstetricians and midwives in hospital delivery teams.

It is referenced, for example, by comedian Dara Ó Briain in his 2010 video *This is the Show*.

- In 2007, The King's Fund found that better cooperation between medical professionals was the single best way to improve outcomes for maternity patients and their babies.

Further reading

Summers A. The mysterious demise of Sarah Gamp: the domiciliary nurse and her detractors, c. 1830–1860. *Victorian Studies.* 1989; **32**(3): 365–86.

7

The 'change': menopause and its meanings

The 'menopause' is essentially a modern concept. It attracted relatively little medical comment before the twentieth century, and, on the few occasions when the end of menstruation was discussed, there was little agreement on its implications for women's ageing. One argument familiar in the Middle Ages held that if menstrual blood was unclean, the woman who no longer underwent periodic purges of such blood was liable to become literally poisoned. Another (broadly Hippocratic) theory was that when women ceased to menstruate, their bodies reverted to being more akin to those of males. This was supposedly a positive attribute, as it implied strength and heightened mental acuity. Throughout recorded history, the process was anticipated to occur by approximately age 55.

After 1900, medicine became more engaged with the topic of menopause, and particularly with hormonal change and the scope for associated therapies. Then in 1949 the French philosopher Simone de Beauvoir published *The Second Sex* and for the first time, menopause was discussed openly in a sociological context. De Beauvoir concentrated on the meanings of the menopause for different types of women but mainly for individuals who subscribed to one of the prevailing models of mid-twentieth-century femininity – namely, the attractive and submissive sexual partner and/or the mother of maturing children. She argued:

> 'The dangerous age' is marked by certain organic disturbances, but what lends them importance is their symbolic significance. The crisis of the 'change of life' is felt much less keenly by women who have not staked everything on their femininity . . .

If women have interests, pursuits or occupations outside of the home and dissociated from home, marriage and family, they will regard the end of menstruation with indifference or relief. For most women, though, the 'crisis' will begin even before hormonal change as they confront the degradation of their facial and bodily appearance. De Beauvoir observes the irony, therefore, that women in their 30s will be witnessing the first discernible decline in their physical attributes at the same time that they reach their sexual peak.

Question: De Beauvoir wrote very frankly about women's sexuality in *The Second Sex*; to what extent did this openness translate to her autobiographical works?

While the 'menopausal' woman is largely absent from historical accounts, the 'lusty widow' is a stereotype that is very familiar from comedic literary texts of the seventeenth century and earlier. Plays and other literary forms depict older women trying to seduce younger men, either with entertaining lack of success or triumph (where the man has an ulterior, often financial, motive). Jennifer Panek, among others, has pointed out that '[n]early all the well-known theatrical names of the first quarter of the seventeenth century produced at least one comic remarrying-widow plot'.

Why is this relevant?

- The sexuality of mature women is still regarded as something of a joke, although cultural interventions such as the television series *Sex in the City* have provided an alternative narrative.
- Despite the advances made by the feminist movement in the second half of the twentieth century, women are often judged primarily on their appearance, age and sexual attractiveness. This makes the loss of looks and fertility a crisis, even when the physiological effects of menopause are muted.
- Women going through the menopause should be advised to avoid weight gain, to exercise, and to not stop having sex.

Further reading

Botelho LA. Old age and menopause in rural women of early modern Suffolk. In: Botelho LA, Thane P, editors. *Women and Ageing in British Society Since 1500*. Harlow: Longman; 2001. pp. 43–65.

de Beauvoir S. *The Second Sex*. London: Jonathan Cape; 1953.

Panek J. *Widows and Suitors in Early Modern English Comedy*. Cambridge: Cambridge University Press; 2004.

Section 4

Infection, immunity and public health

1

The 'king's evil' or 'wasting disease': tuberculosis

What do the following people have in common?
- Emily Bronte
- Florence Nightingale
- John Keats
- George Orwell
- Nelson Mandela
- Tom Jones

They all suffered and/or died from tuberculosis.

This disease has been often romanticised in literature, film and music. Many heroes and heroines have succumbed to pulmonary tuberculosis, also dubbed 'consumption' or 'phthisis', including Mimi in Puccini's opera *La bohème* (1896), Fantine in Victor Hugo's novel *Les Misérables* (1862) and Satine in Baz Luhrmann's film *Moulin Rouge!* (2001). Its aesthetic appeal may have related to its propensity to affect young people without destroying appearance or causing too much pain:

> General emaciation takes place, the cheek bones are prominent, the eyes hollow and languid ... Still, however, the appearance often remains good, and the patient has a craving for solid food, from which circumstance he is likely to flatter himself with a speedy recovery ...
>
> R Thomas, *A Treatise on Domestic Medicine*, 1822: 286

In fact, the nineteenth-century image of female beauty came to be shaped by the physical effects of consumption, as can be seen in the Pre-Raphaelite paintings of thin pale heroines with flushed cheeks. Lord Byron allegedly declared a wish to die with consumption because the ladies would comment on 'how interesting he looks in dying'. Consumption was considered a mark of the creative personality – particularly since so many brilliant and creative talents became its victims. According to Alexander Dumas, 'in 1823 and 1824 it was the fashion to suffer from the lungs'. This was the Romantic age that saw beauty in corruption. The reality, especially for the poor, was very different.

There was little understanding of the cause of consumption until the germ theory of disease was accepted (*see* Chapter 4 in this section, 'Germ theory'). Its infectivity had been observed by the Arabic physician Avicenna (980–1037 AD) in the eleventh century AD, who introduced quarantine. In 1546, a physician and Paduan professor Girolamo Fracastoro (1478–1553) wrote *De Contagione* [On contagion], in which he included 'physis' and described his theory that epidemic diseases were spread by direct or indirect contact with 'spores' rather than 'miasma' (bad air); however, it is unclear whether he considered these to be microorganisms or chemicals. In contrast, in 1722, the instrument-maker Benjamin Martin, in his book, *A New Theory of Consumption* referred to 'animaliculae or their seed – inimical to our Nature [transmitted by] a Breath [that a consumptive] emits from his Lungs . . . that might be caught by a sound Person'. His account was proved over 100 years later by a French army physician, Jean Antoine Villemin (1827–92). In 1865, Villemin inoculated rabbits with material from infected humans and cattle, which then became infected; his discovery was initially ignored. This may have been because other views about its aetiology were preferred – in particular, the idea that some people had a hereditary weakness for the illness. This must have seemed plausible, given that often many generations of the same family were affected. Further, authorities like Sir James Clark (1788–1870), a physician to Queen Victoria, completely rejected that it was contagious in his *Treatise on Pulmonary Consumption: comprehending an inquiry into the causes, nature, prevention, and treatment of tuberculous and scrofulous diseases in general* of 1835. Some of the orthodox explanations are well illustrated by this extract from Dr Thomas' *Domestic Medicine* of 1822:

> [I]ts frequency in Great Britain may be attributed principally to the variableness of the climate, sudden transitions from heat to cold . . .
>
> I look upon the application of cold united to moisture, as by lying on a damp bed, wearing wet clothes . . . to be the most exciting cause of pulmonary consumption, this giving rise to catarrh . . . which ultimately terminates in the formation of an abscess or in causing tubercles . . . [T]he dust to which certain artificers are exposed, as millers, stone cutters, bakers, hairdressers . . . are likewise to be looked upon as causes . . .
>
> Consumption is ever to be considered as a very dangerous disease, but still most so when arriving from an hereditary predisposition . . . (287)

Theories on what caused the illness influenced management. Many thought the disease could be reversed if caught in its latent phase or even prevented, so advocated a change of climate. For some time, a mild climate was considered best, which is why the poet John Keats was sent to Italy where he got worse and died. In 1840, an English country physician, George Bodington (1799–1882), published *On the Treatment and Cure of Pulmonary Consumption*, in which he advocated fresh air, sun, exercise and good nutrition, but his views were firmly dismissed by one reviewer (*Lancet*. 1839: **40**(ii):p 575.) who thought there was no point in 'expending any portion of our critical wrath on his crude ideas and unsupported assertion'. However, another advocate, Hermann Brehmer (1826–89), established the first sanatorium in 1859 at Görbersdorf, Silesia, with a strict regime of exposure to fresh air, exercise and good diet. One of his former patients, an army surgeon, founded his own sanatorium near Frankfurt in 1876 but replaced exercise with strict rest. In the USA, Edward Trudeau (1848–1915) established a very popular sanatorium in the Adirondack mountains in the early 1880s, where one of his early patients was Robert Louis Stevenson, the author of *Treasure Island*. Gradually, the sanatorium movement expanded across all of Europe, including Britain, reaching its peak by the beginning of the First World War.

Once the infective nature of tuberculosis was acknowledged and the causative bacillus identified, significant public health measures were taken. Public education was used to prevent spread of infection, spitting was discouraged and hygiene taught in schools. Advertisements appeared on buses and hoardings designed to convince the public of the infective nature of tuberculosis. Town planners were asked to provide open spaces to ensure ready access to fresh air. Legislation was introduced to support public health measures, such as ensuring that herds were tuberculin tested and milk certified; this led to the virtual disappearance of infected neck glands in children. In 1899, voluntary notification of cases was introduced in Britain, followed by mandatory notification of all cases by 1911. The National Insurance Act 1911 required free home treatment by panel doctors and local-authority spending on sanatoriums and research. Voluntary dispensaries were established that housed patients waiting to enter a sanatorium. In the 1940s, to reduce infection in the workplace, maintenance allowances were given to infected workers, who were usually the main breadwinners, when they stopped working to undergo treatment.

When Robert Koch (1843–1910) identified the tuberculosis bacillus in 1882, there were hopes that an immunising agent would soon follow (*see* Chapter 3 in this section, 'From variolation to vaccination'). Unfortunately 'tuberculin', a glycerine extract of the bacillus, failed to be an effective vaccine. However, it did turn out to be a useful diagnostic tool, because it caused an allergic reaction in people who had been previously exposed to the tuberculosis bacillus.

Question 1: What was the medical significance of having a diagnostic test?

The chest X-ray proved to be another very useful epidemiological tool, which was extensively used for testing soldiers in both world wars and people in the workplace. Suspicion of any infection could be followed up with bacteriological testing. At last, René Laennec's (1781–1826) identification of pathological lesions in the chest through using mediate auscultation and the stethoscope was now being visualised (*see* Section 6, Chapter 3, 'The rise of modern medicine: the evolution of physical diagnosis').

Apart from staying in a sanatorium, which only the wealthy could afford to do in the nineteenth century, historic treatments were limited. Up until the early eighteenth century, a widely observed ritual in both France and England was that of obtaining the king's touch to cure tubercular adenitis, also known as 'scrofula'. Scrofula, although unsightly, often remits spontaneously. Serendipitous remission together with alms (a coin was often given to the individual which came to be known as the 'king's penny') must have consolidated the royal reputation. The following is a literary account of the ritual:

> [S]trangely visited people,
> All swoln and ulcerous, pitiful to the eye
> The mere despair of surgery, he cures,
> Hanging a golden stamp about their necks,
> Put on with holy prayers: and 'tis spoken,
> To the succeeding royalty he leaves
> The healing benediction.

> Shakespeare, *Macbeth*, Act 4, Scene 3, lines 150–6

In contrast to this benign quackery, the 'plombage' technique was dramatic and risky. The Italian physician Carlo Forlanini (1847–1918) had observed that when tubercular sufferers experienced a spontaneous pneumothorax, their prognosis improved. In 1906, he published his account of a technique to artificially induce a pneumothorax using small incremental injections of nitrous oxide to compress and collapse the lung. The rationale was that the tubercular lesions would be more likely to heal in a resting lung. Some lungs would not collapse because of adhesions. A surgical technique was soon developed to cut them using an instrument inserted in the chest wall. Subsequently, 'thoracoplasty' was introduced, which entailed removing rib segments, but this caused irreversible deformity. Although artificially induced pneumothorax continued to be used until the late 1940s, there was no evidence that it was effective.

In the meantime, despite Koch's difficulties with tuberculin, an effective vaccine was developed in 1924 at the Pasteur Institute by Albert Calmette (1863–1933) and Camille Guérin (1872–1961) that they called 'Vaccin Bilié de Calmette et Guérin' and which was commonly known as 'BCG'. It was soon widely used, but there was significant controversy about it after several babies died following the vaccination; however, it was shown that the vaccine had been contaminated in the cases that had proved fatal. By 1950, most European countries including Britain as well as countries in North Africa, the Middle East, South Asia and some in South America had adopted a mass immunisation programme.

Treatment for those already infected was slower to reach fruition. Streptomycin was first introduced in the mid-1940s but resistant strains limited its efficacy. Para-aminosalicylic acid and isoniazid followed, which, in combination with streptomycin, could treat most cases of pulmonary tuberculosis.

From the 1750s to the late nineteenth century, tuberculosis was hugely prevalent, reaching epidemic proportions in Europe and America. At least one in eight deaths in Britain was due to the disease. Population increase and mass urbanisation no doubt contributed to its ubiquity. By 1987, there were only 5000 cases per year in the UK. Since then, the rate has risen, particularly in underdeveloped and poorer countries, but also in the big cities of major European countries. In 1993, the WHO declared a global health emergency because of the resurgence of tuberculosis.

Question 2: Why has the prevalence of tuberculosis increased so much over the last three decades?

Why is this relevant?

- Public health measures are just as important now as in the past.
- The poor, homeless and immunosuppressed continue to be at most risk of contracting tuberculosis.
- Although we now understand the causes of the disease, we are still chasing treatments that work as the bacillus becomes drug resistant.
- To successfully control tuberculosis in the past, many different agencies, disciplines and countries had to collaborate. This lesson is still pertinent today.

Further reading

Bynum H. *Spitting Blood: the history of tuberculosis*. Oxford: Oxford University Press; 2012.

Cronin AJ. *The Citadel* [novel] London: Back Bay; 1983.

Sakula A. Carlo Foralnini, inventor of artificial pneumothorax for the treatment of pulmonary tuberculosis. *Thorax*. 1983; **38**(5): 326–32.

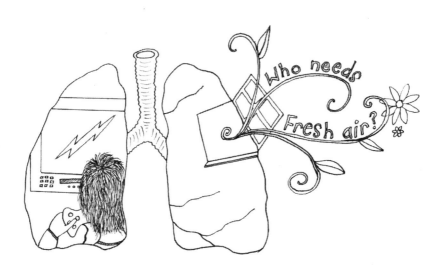

2

Health and livelihood

ILL-HEALTH HAS TRADITIONALLY HAD A DRAMATIC IMPACT ON PEOPLE'S ability to earn a living. For many ordinary working people at most points in the past, ill-health or injury that prevented people from working meant a reduction or loss of earnings *and* increased outgoings in relation to medicines, medical attendance or nursing care. Towards the end of the seventeenth century, recognition of this double-bind encouraged the founding of 'friendly societies', also known as 'box clubs'. These clubs were funded by member contributions and offered payments in cases of unemployment from ill-health, age or disability. They also pledged to meet members' funeral expenses. Clubs might be based around communities, congregations, workplaces or employment sectors. At first, they tended to be short-lived; club treasurers were lay people without significant financial experience and typically funds were lost (through actuarial incompetence or embezzlement). Eventually, the societies became better run and more robust, and some societies became affiliated to one another. The most prominent included the Independent Order of Odd Fellows and the Ancient Order of Foresters. Millions of working-class men were members of friendly societies by the end of the nineteenth century, but they were only ever the preserve of workers who could afford the contributions.

In the twentieth century, National Insurance began to provide a measure of security for working people. The National Insurance Act 1911 enforced contributions from employers and the state, in addition to employees, to fund 15 weeks of employment benefit to unemployed shipbuilders, engineering workers and building workers. Subsequent acts extended the benefits to employees of other sectors and increased the duration of payments but did not tackle the issue of paying for illness or injury.

The challenge of meeting costs of medical goods and services has been mitigated (but not erased) in England since the introduction of the NHS in 1948 and the provision for medical attention to be free at the first point of contact (although prescription and other charges have been a constant feature of the system). Risks of income reduction are still heavily dependent on the practices of employers. Some professional workers are able to fall ill and be absent from work for 6 months or more while remaining on full pay. Others in the unskilled labouring workforce – for example, in the building trades – may only be entitled to Statutory Sick Pay or minimal benefits. Financial difficulties multiply in households in which there is only one breadwinner who becomes chronically ill or incapacitated.

> **Question 1**: Consult and compare two websites representing two different types of employee: the Union of Construction, Allied Trades and Technicians (www.ucatt. org.uk/) and the British Medical Association (bma.org.uk/).
> How does each body deal with the issue of sick pay? What is the difference in the treatment of the topic between the two?
>
> **Question 2**: Now consult the two websites to compare the two different sectors of employment in terms of risks to employees. Builders and doctors are both exposed to work-related hazards but of different kinds.
> What is the mid- to long-term employment/earnings outlook for a builder with a musculoskeletal disorder, as opposed to a doctor who contracts hepatitis B? In either case, has the outlook changed recently?

Numerous factors contribute to the fact that healthcare workers are much better placed to manage the economic problems associated with periods of ill-health than construction workers in twenty-first century Britain.

British government intervention in the field of workplace insecurity is delivered via the benefits system, but this does not necessarily mitigate the penalties of temporary injury or long-term disability. A historic tendency to view all welfare systems as open to abuse encourages cyclical insistence on policing benefit claimants and their justifications for assistance, on the grounds that any form of support may operate as a disincentive to self-help. This was the case in 1834 (with the implementation of the Poor Law Amendment Act, imposing stringent requirements on anyone so poor they could not make ends meet without aid) and was echoed as recently as 2012 with the introduction of new barriers to claimants of the Disability Living Allowance (*see* Section 5, Chapter 2, 'Two steps forward, one step back: disability'). In such circumstances, the imposition of requirements to prove eligibility *may* assist in removing the 'undeserving' from the list of recipients, but it *certainly* has a punitive effect on all applicants. Further, such barriers have the unintended consequence of inhibiting or preventing valid claims from being submitted, because those with physical ill-health are unnecessarily distressed by the need to prove entitlement, while those with mental ill-health may find it impossible to demonstrate.

Why is this relevant?

- Illness and injury, and consequential entitlement to sick pay or access to state benefits, can play an enormous part in people's attitude towards their health and their tendency to either seek medical assistance or avoid it.
- Most people are not very well protected against the economic decline inherent in failing health.

- Medical professionals are at particular risk of encountering, for example, infectious disease, but are rarely subject to indirect penalties for contracting them via work.
- The risk that infectious disease will have a serious impact on medical professionals and their ability to pursue their livelihood is relatively remote.
- Not all first-world countries protect their workers in the same ways as Britain – most notably the USA, where the concept of 'socialised medicine' is a source of much political disagreement and economic opposition (not least from the entrenched private medical insurance lobby). This leaves some workers particularly vulnerable in an otherwise-wealthy nation.

Further reading

Cordery S. *British Friendly Societies, 1750–1914*. Basingstoke: Palgrave Macmillan; 2003.
Gosden PHJH. *The Friendly Societies in England, 1815–1875*. Manchester: Manchester University Press; 1961.
www.bma.org.uk
www.ucatt.info

3

From variolation to vaccination

[T]he sick and the dying were tended by pitying care of those who had recovered, because they knew the course of the disease and were free of apprehension. For no one was ever attacked a second time, or not with a fatal result.

Thucydides on immunity, History of the Peloponnesian War, 430 BC

THUS, THUCYDIDES (c. 460–c. 395 BC), WHO IS SOMETIMES REFERRED TO as the first scientific historian, realised that plague survivors were immune to reinfection from a deadly disease that had killed 30 000 people. Centuries later, it became common practice in some cultures to protect people from infectious disease by artificial induction of immunity, although without any knowledge of how this worked. The earliest written accounts of inoculation are possibly in an eighth-century medical Buddhist text called the *Nidana* from India. By the sixteenth century, the Chinese were practising nose insufflation using silver blowpipes containing powdered smallpox pustules taken only from people who seemed not to be severely infected. The practice of inoculation, or 'variolation', was disseminated to Europe through a physician, Emmanuel Timoni (c. 1670–1718), who had encountered it in Constantinople where infected smallpox material was taken from pustules and transferred to an area of scratched skin of the person to be inoculated for the purposes of immunisation. He wrote a letter published in *Philosophical Transactions of the Royal Society of Medicine* in 1714 that was read by two people who would proceed to pioneer it: a Bostonian clergyman, Cotton Mather (1663–1728), and the wife of the British ambassador to the Ottoman Empire, Lady Mary Wortley Montagu (1689–1762).

In 1713, there had been another outbreak of smallpox on the east coast of colonial America. This disease was a serious threat to settlers and had devastated the Native Americans who had had no previous exposure to the disease, so had not acquired any immunity. Mather allegedly knew from a Sudanese slave that inoculation was practised in Africa, so Timoni's account was not a great surprise. Thus, when smallpox reappeared in 1721 carried by a ship from the West Indies, Mather urged local physicians to try the method. Dr Zabdiel Boylston agreed to inoculate his only son and his two slaves who all recovered. But the intervention proved to be enormously controversial, both with the medical fraternity and the clergy, who asserted that it was against the will of God.

Lady Montagu had witnessed the practice for herself while living in Istanbul. Her brother had died of the disease and she had been disfigured. She was sufficiently persuaded to ask Charles Maitland (1668–1748), who had been the embassy physician in Constantinople, to inoculate her son. Later, she had her daughter inoculated and publicised its benefits to the English aristocracy. Maitland asked permission of the royal family to experiment on some condemned prisoners at Newgate Prison. The prisoners survived and were set free in exchange for their cooperation. It was then tried on six orphans with success. As a result, King George I allowed two of his grandchildren to be inoculated. However, just as in Boston, there was considerable opposition from the medical and ecclesiastical establishment, and some of the medical concerns were justified, as the procedure was not completely safe; inoculation caused death in 2%–3% of cases. Yet the risks were far greater from smallpox, which accounted for 20% of all deaths in the eighteenth and early nineteenth centuries and caused significant disfigurement among survivors.

Variolation became popular in England but other countries were not so keen. The French Enlightenment philosopher and satirist Voltaire (1694–1778) remarks in his book *Letters on England* of 1731 how the English were regarded by the rest of Christian Europe as 'fools and madmen' for their habit of inoculating their children. He praises Lady Montagu for championing the custom, thereby saving so many lives, and opines that the French 'are an odd kind of people. Perhaps our nation will imitate ten years hence this practice of the English, if the clergy and physicians will give them leave to do'. Over the following years, the procedure became much safer in England, thanks to an approach used by the surgeon Robert Sutton. Although Sutton kept his methods secret to deter competitors, his son revealed in the 1770s what the key points of their approach were: the use of mildly affected donors, shallow scratches and no bleeding.

> **Discussion point**:
> In 2012, students at a college in Austin, Texas refused to enrol because of a strict vaccination requirement, as attested by a headline at the time: 'Anti vaccine backlash: thousands refuse to enroll in Austin Community College' (C Stellpflag, NaturalNews.com [website], 25 May 2012). What contemporary arguments have been raised against vaccination?

The 1853 Vaccination Act required vaccination against smallpox for all infants in the first 3 months of their life. What had changed over the previous 50 years to prompt the usually liberal British to pass such intrusive legislation?

Vaccination was not the same as variolation. It was popularised by Edward Jenner (1749–1823), who conferred scientific status on the intervention, yet was not the first to discover it. Jenner's experiments occurred 22 years after Benjamin Jesty (c. 1736–1816), a farmer, observed the protective effects of cowpox infection among milkmaids. He persuaded his wife and their two sons to be inoculated with cowpox, which he did using a stocking needle. In 1798, Jenner published a book, *An Inquiry into the Causes and Effects of Variolae Vaccinae or Cowpox* describing his theory of why cowpox could protect against smallpox and his results on subjects he had inoculated with scabs from people infected with cowpox; these subjects subsequently recovered quickly from deliberate exposure to smallpox. He called the process 'vaccination' because the immunising material was from cows (and *vacca* is the Latin for cow). In 1801, Jenner observed:

> The numbers who have partaken of its benefits throughout Europe and other parts of the globe are incalculable; ... the annihilation of smallpox, the most dreadful scourge of the human species, must be the final result of this practice.

Vaccination with cowpox proved to be much safer than variolation, which was made illegal in Britain in 1840. Nonetheless, the 1853 act was perceived as an infringement of civil liberties and incited significant hostility. Corruption was suspected, as vaccine manufacturers made huge profits. Anti-vaccination demonstrations occurred and concerns were raised about the safety and efficacy of the vaccine. Nevertheless, a further act was passed in 1873, strengthening the compulsory nature of vaccination, although by the end of the century administrative difficulties in claiming conscientious exemption were removed. The government entirely removed required vaccination in 1946.

Question 1: In 2010, a blog post titled 'MMR-autism scare: so, farewell then, Dr Andrew Wakefield' (T Chivers, [blog post], *The Telegraph*, 24 May) was published. Wakefield's research concluded that there was a link between the measles, mumps and rubella (MMR) vaccine and autism and bowel disease. What damage did Wakefield's fraudulent research do?

Jenner was fortunate enough to have come across a pox virus – cowpox – that conferred immunity against another type of pox virus – smallpox. This situation is really quite unusual; most future vaccines would need to contain a dead or attenuated pathogen in order to confer immunity. Louis Pasteur (1822–95) encountered the phenomenon of the power of the attenuated vaccine when he found that inoculation with germs causing cholera in 2-week-old chickens induced protection against younger virulent germs. Modern vaccination methodology was developed by Pasteur through application of his knowledge of Jenner's procedures to his own observations. Pasteur's and his colleagues' legacy was the development of a number of vaccines against major infectious diseases.

Question 2: Between 1885 and 1897, vaccines were developed for seven major infectious diseases. What were these?

Why is this relevant?

- The last 150 years have seen the eradication of many major causes of mortality through vaccination programmes. Their efficacy can be undermined by poor public take-up. This raises the question of whether vaccination programmes should be made mandatory.
- Concerns exist now about bioterrorism. Should we keep the smallpox virus to manufacture vaccine in case the virus is 'manufactured' by terrorists? Indeed, should we vaccinate key personnel with smallpox vaccine?
- We are annually faced with the challenge of developing vaccines for new strains of influenza virus that now spread with a rapidity unknown before air travel.
- Pasteur's insights could not have happened without other technological and conceptual developments. (To discover more, *see* the next chapter, 'The germ theory of disease'.)
- Programmes of vaccination continue to be threatened by non-scientific ideologies. In December 2012, the Islamic fundamentalist group the Taliban claimed that polio vaccine altered children's DNA thereby making them infertile and halted the vaccination programme in Pakistan by murdering some of the vaccinators.

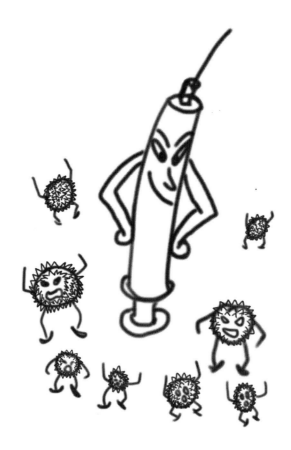

Further reading

Bardell D. Nestling cuckoos to vaccination: a commemoration of Edward Jenner. *BioScience.* 1996; **46**(11): 866–71.

Durbach N. *Bodily Matters: the anti-vaccination movement in England, 1853–1907.* Durham, NC: Duke University Press; 2005.

Mercer AJ. Smallpox and epidemic-demographical–demographic change in Europe: the role of vaccination. *Population Studies.* 1985; **39**(2): 287–307.

Razzell PE. *The Conquest of Smallpox: the impact of inoculation on smallpox mortality in eighteenth century Britain.* 2nd ed. London: Caliban; 2003.

Williams G. *Angel of Death: the story of smallpox.* Basingstoke: Palgrave Macmillan; 2010.

Wolfe RM, Sharp LK. Anti-vaccinationists, past and present. *British Medical Journal.* 2002; **325**(7361): 430–2.

4

The germ theory of disease

[I]n swampy places minute creatures live which float in the air that cannot be discerned with the eye and enter the body through the mouth and nostrils and there cause serious disease . . .

Marcus Terentius Varro, *De Re Rustica* [On Agriculture], 36 BC

THE IDEA THAT LIVING ENTITIES TOO SMALL TO SEE CAN CAUSE DISEASE seems obvious to us, yet Varro's (116–27 BC) insight was to take at least another 1800 years to prove. In 1546, Girolamo Fracastoro speculated in his publication *De Contagione* that disease was caused by disease 'spores', which could be carried by human contact or the wind, but he did not have a microscope to demonstrate such small entities. In contrast, knowledge started to develop about the parasite. The 1491 edition of *The Great Herball* has possibly the first illustrations of parasites and the *Boke of Husbandrye* published in 1523 by Sir Anthony Fitzherbert contains a description of the liver fluke. But lay people mostly believed in various – now apprehended as imaginary – agents of disease such as the 'wyrm'. There was thought to be, for example, a hand-wyrm, a fic-wyrm (which caused piles), a smea-wyrm of ulcers, a tooth-wyrm of tooth decay and a heart wyrm, which caused sudden death.

Whether agents of disease could be seen or not, it was widely believed that they were spontaneously generated within the body by some mysterious process. The Aristotelian belief that living things could emerge from non-living things did much to inhibit investigation of how diseases could be transmitted or managed. It continued to be accepted dogma, despite experimental challenges in 1668 by a physician, Francesco Redi (1626–97) and a century later by a Catholic priest and physiologist Lazzaro Spallanzani (1729–99).

Two particular developments helped to undermine the doctrine, one technical and one conceptual. First, in the 1670s, Antonie van Leeuwenhoek (1632–1723) created lenses that could magnify up to 200 times. During his life, he discovered bacteria, cell vacuoles and spermatozoa using his microscopes. He was made a fellow of the Royal Society of London, with which he maintained a long correspondence. A contemporary, Robert Hooke (1635–1703), curator of experiments at the Royal Society, published *Micrographia* in 1665 and is often considered to be

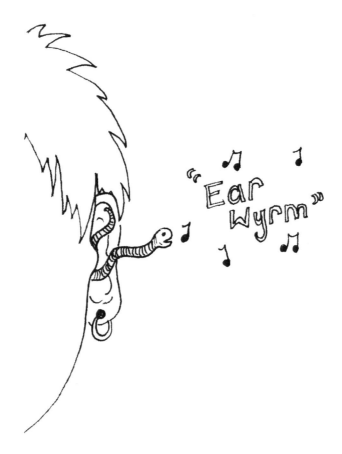

the father of microscopy for his detailed illustrations; however, microscopy could not improve until the problem of chromatic distortion was solved (*see* Section 6, Chapter 5, 'From toy to tool: the microscope').

Then, in the seventeenth century, English physician Thomas Sydenham (1624–89), introduced the idea that each disease was identifiable through the symptoms and signs it produced. His process of classification is essentially the one used in modern medicine. This notion of specificity of disease was further developed by Pierre-Fidèle Bretonneau (1778–1862), who thought that each disease had a unique cause. In 1840, Jakob Henle (1809–85), a physician and physiologist from Zurich, argued in 'On miasma and contagion' that the difference between infectious diseases was due to different living causal agents.

The stage was now set for Louis Pasteur's (1822–95) work on fermentation and the development of a coherent germ theory. Between 1860 and 1864, Pasteur demonstrated that microorganisms are present in the air and responsible for disease, infection, fermentation and putrefaction. He showed that specific diseases were caused by particular microorganisms and he developed vaccines, which gave protection against rabies and anthrax. The German physician Robert Koch

(1843–1910) conclusively proved the germ theory of disease in his paper 'The aetiology of traumatic infective diseases' first published in 1878. In this paper, he laid down four conditions or postulates by which a bacterium could be proven to cause a specific condition. He developed solid media for growing pure cultures of bacteria easily and recognised that methyl violet dye could show up the bacillus responsible for septicaemia. His methods were used to discover the causal agents for diphtheria, typhoid, gonorrhoea, leprosy, tetanus, plague, syphilis, whooping cough and streptococcal and staphylococcal infections.

Question: What are Koch's postulates?

Why is this relevant?

- The rejection of the doctrine of spontaneous generation and proof of germ theory is arguably the single most important concept in public health and modern medicine.
- The global resurgence of infectious diseases such as tuberculosis and new strains of influenza virus ensures this discovery remains highly relevant.
- Joseph Lister's awareness of Pasteur's experiments led him to appreciate how wound sepsis could occur. As a result, he tried to create, with the use of carbolic spray, antiseptic conditions at the wound site. His methods, which were initially met with hostility from the surgical community, were gradually accepted thanks to a proven rationale. In time, a shift in approach occurred to the use of aseptic techniques in order to prevent the presence of any offending microorganisms. Although Lister was not the first to introduce this, he later became an advocate. Consequently, the risks of surgery significantly reduced and the speciality was transformed (*see* Section 7, Chapter 6, 'Cutting for the stone: the hazards of surgery').

Further reading

Nuland SB. *The Doctors' Plague: germs, childbed fever, and the strange story of Ignáz Semmelweis*. New York, NY: WW Norton; 2004.

Pasteur L, Lister J. *Germ Theory and its Applications to Medicine and on the Antiseptic Principle of the Practice of Surgery*. New York, NY: Prometheus; 1996.

5

Syphilis, self-pollution and stigma

GONORRHOEA HAS BEEN PRESENT IN HUMAN POPULATIONS FOR thousands of years, whereas syphilis was unknown until the late fifteenth century. The first outbreak of syphilis is thought to have occurred in the 1490s among a group of European soldiers. In its earliest epidemics, syphilis proved highly virulent and could kill sufferers quite quickly. The symptoms comprised irritating pustules on the genitals, where scratching soon lead to ulceration. A contemporary who contracted the disease in 1498, Joseph Grunpeck, has left us this description of his sufferings: 'The disease loosed its first arrow into my priapic glans which, on account of the wound, became so swollen that both hands could scarcely circle it' (Quetel C. *History of Syphilis*. Baltimore: Johns Hopkins University Press. 1990).

As syphilis became endemic in European society, it developed three phases recognised by contemporaries. The first phase involving visible ulceration of the genitals was succeeded by a second phase often characterised by a rash. The latent period that followed might last for decades (and was not understood as an additional phase); it is likely that a significant proportion of the European population became infected with syphilis, perhaps up to 10%, but that latency encouraged people to think that they were cured. People who lived long enough suffered a third phase. The neurosyphilitic variety can present with insidious changes to the personality, mood disorder, psychotic symptoms, dementia and a singular type of gait called 'tabes dorsalis' – collectively, these symptoms are called 'general paralysis of the insane'. A more benign version presents with hideous lesions called 'gumma', which can occur on the face and are particularly stigmatising. (For the treatment of syphilis with mercury, *see* Section 7, Chapter 1, 'The appeal of the miracle cure').

Question: What has syphilis colloquially been known as in the past? What does this suggest about the potentially stigmatising nature of an obvious diagnosis?

Syphilis is typically contracted via sexual intercourse (although it can also be carried by shared blood, so can be transmitted to infants in utero via the placenta). Sheldon Watts argues that attitudes to sex in general and masturbation in particular contributed significantly to the prevalence of syphilis in the eighteenth and nineteenth centuries. Masturbation or 'self-abuse' was thought to be a direct cause of mental aberration and insanity as well as theologically wicked. As such, any publications treating the topic depicted it as highly damaging and significantly worse for both body and soul than seeking sexual gratification outside of marriage. The treatise *Onania; Or, the Heinous Sin of Self Pollution, And All Its Frightful Consequences, In Both Sexes, Considered: With Spiritual and Physical Advice to Those Who have Already Injured Themselves By this Abominable Practice* by Dutch theologian Dr Balthazar Bekker was first published in England around 1710, for example, and contributed significantly to this point of view. In such an intellectual environment, prostitution became an unfortunate necessity and widespread syphilis infection an unintended consequence.

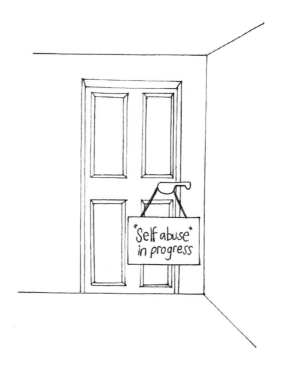

Syphilis also supplies an instance of the most grotesque exploitation of a patient population by medical research. In Tuskegee, Alabama, a programme of research investigated the presentation of untreated syphilis in black men. The study achieved its ends by apparently offering the men free healthcare, but in fact delivering no recognised treatment for syphilis. Indeed, researchers concealed the diagnosis from the study's patients and did not tell them about the development of penicillin as a viable cure for their complaint. The study ran from 1932 for 40 years and involved around 600 men. The ethical failings of the study, and particularly its wilful failure to treat its participants, were eventually exposed by the newspapers, and the resulting scandal gave rise to changes in American law and a much greater measure of protection for patients in trials. However, the lengthy duration of the study meant that action was only taken after some of the men's wives had been infected and some of their children had been born with congenital syphilis.

The first effective anti-syphilitic drug that did not contain mercury was developed in the first decade of the twentieth century and was marketed from 1910 as Salvarsan. Even so, general paralysis of the insane continued to be given as a cause of death in Britain into the 1920s.

Why is this relevant?

- Sexual disease has been historically stigmatising because it has implied promiscuity and sin (albeit a lesser sin than masturbation).
- Sexuality, secrecy and stigma are not confined to the period before 1900; in the late twentieth century, human immunodeficiency virus (HIV) became such a source of concern for public health that government-sponsored advertisements were screened on television warning the British population about the risks of unprotected sex with a person who carried the infection.
- The prevalence of syphilis is rising again but now in the developing world, especially in Sub-Saharan Africa. It is often associated with HIV. There are various reasons why prevalence has increased in recent decades but one is unsafe sexual practices, especially in Catholic countries in which prophylactic contraception is technically forbidden on doctrinal grounds. The victims are not just adults but also the children of affected mothers.

Further reading

Hayden D. *Pox: genius, madness and the mysteries of syphilis.* New York, NY: Basic; 2004.

Watts S. *Epidemics and History: disease, power and imperialism.* New Haven, CT: Yale University Press; 1997.

6

'Flu pandemics of the twentieth century

I had a little bird,
Its name was Enza,
I opened the window,
And in-flu-enza.

Children's skipping rhyme, 1918

AS THE FIRST WORLD WAR WAS ENDING IN 1918, A 'FLU PANDEMIC rapidly spread around the world, probably as a result of the massive demobilisation of soldiers. It was called the 'Spanish 'flu' because of the exceptionally high rate of mortality in Spain earlier in the same year, where 8 million people died. Although 35 to 50 million people are estimated to have died in total, it is likely that this is a conservative calculation and some argue that the mortality figure was twice this. This means that in 1918–19, more people died in 1 year than in the 4 years of the Black Death from 1347 to 1351. The 'flu was totally lethal in pregnant women, and all adults aged 20–40 years were particularly vulnerable. The mortality rate was higher in poor countries such as India and in the army camps than it was elsewhere in the developed world. A day nurse working at Camp Humphries in Virginia wrote to her friend:

> When I was in the Officer's barracks, four officers whom I had charge of, died. Two of them were married and called for their wife nearly all the time. It was sure pitiful to see them die. I was right in the wards alone with them each time and Oh! The first one that died sure unnerved me.
>
> … Orderlies carried dead soldiers out on stretchers at a rate of two every three hours.
>
> www.archives.gov/exhibits/influenza-epidemic/recordslist-htlm
> (accessed 3 May 2013)

The public health response was slow but, once mobilised, included a variety of measures based on an understanding of the germ theory of disease infectivity (*see* Chapter 4 in this section, 'The germ theory of disease). Acknowledgement that the offending microbe spread through air droplets led to restrictions on, or banning of, public gatherings at venues such as dance halls and cinemas. People were encouraged to walk to work to avoid poorly ventilated and crowded buses. Institutional quarantine occurred in the military camps. In the USA, posters appeared educating the public on respiratory hygiene, hand washing and the use of common crockery. Gauze masks were encouraged and even required in some states, but there was a significant shortage of these. The following ditty was constructed to remind the public: 'Obey the laws, And wear the gauze, / Protect your jaws, From septic paws' (virus.stanford.edu/uda/fluresponse.html (accessed 3 May 2013)).

Preventative measures and diagnostic acumen were more sophisticated than treatment at this time; however, the pandemic galvanised clinicians and scientists to find the causative agent. Thanks to a newly developed investigative procedure of taking samples of sputum and blood for culture, it became possible to isolate the causative microorganism, which turned out to be not a bacillus but a virus. Culturing was made possible due to the invention of the Petri dish by Julius Richard Petri (1852–1921), an assistant to the German physician Robert Koch (1843–1910), one of the main proponents of microbiology.

Question: What was it now theoretically possible to achieve?

There were to be another four pandemics over the ensuing 90 years due to *Influenza A virus* subtypes. The first of these was Asian 'flu in 1957–58, which was due the human form of H2N2 combining with a mutant strain from ducks. Of those who developed viral pneumonia, 25% died and about 2 million people in total died; especially vulnerable were older people. In 1968–69, 1 million people died as a result of the Hong Kong 'flu, which was due to H3N2; again, older people were particularly at risk. Then, in 1997, the bird 'flu pandemic, due to H5N1, struck. This spread from poultry to humans. More recently, the swine flu pandemic of 2009 resulted in 18 000 deaths. This 'flu was due to a new strain of H1N1 that originated in Mexico and spread from pigs. On 25 April 2009, the WHO declared this outbreak a public health emergency of international concern. By June, it was considered a global pandemic. Eighty-five per cent of the poorest countries could not afford to buy vaccine. Nine countries promised to release 10% of their vaccine stock to the WHO. Only six pharmaceutical companies agreed to do the same.

Why is this relevant?

- It seems that the media is preoccupied with the prospect of a global catastrophe derived from epidemic infection. This century and the last have witnessed a number of books, television series and films on the subject of an apocalypse due to a pernicious microorganism such as:

- *The Scarlet Plague* (1912) by Jack London: a novel set in San Francisco in 2072, 60 years after a plague has depopulated the planet.
- *The Stand* (1978) by Stephen King: an influenza pandemic wipes out most of the global population in this novel.
- *Survivors* (1970s, remade 2008): a television series about a genetically engineered virus.
- *Plague Year* trilogy (2007–9) by Jeff Carlson: in these novels, a nanotech contagion has devoured all warm-blooded life.

● This is not a new phenomenon; Mary Shelley's book of 1826, *The Last Man*, describes a world in the future emptied by a plague. However, today's public has higher expectations of our healthcare systems and news travels instantaneously. Healthcare professionals are expected to be knowledgeable and responsive to the latest pandemic fear. Public health specialists have the responsibility of advising government on effective and efficient measures and the public expects the government to pay the cost of protecting its citizens. The public and media in the UK have alternately criticised the government for being either lackadaisical or over-cautious during recent 'flu scares.

● Public health medicine declined in the second half of the last century, especially following apparent successes in eradicating a number of contagious diseases. However, with the recrudescence of tuberculosis (*see* Chapter 1 in this section, 'The "king's evil" or "wasting disease": tuberculosis') and concerns about influenza pandemics, it has regained its importance.

● There are serious ethical issues to be resolved about the global distribution of vaccines; otherwise, economically poorer countries will suffer most.

Further reading

Barry JM. *The Great Influenza: the story of the deadliest pandemic in history.* London: Penguin; 2005.

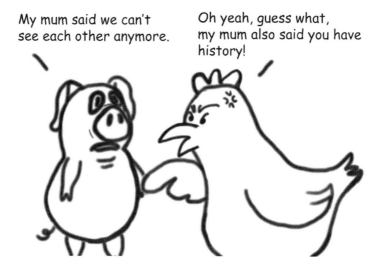

7

Child welfare

DAVID ROWLAND WORKED AS A PIECER AT A TEXTILE MILL IN Manchester. He was interviewed by Michael Sadler and his House of Commons Committee on 10 July 1832:

Q: At what age did you commence working in a cotton mill? A: Just when I had turned six.

Q: What employment had you in a mill in the first instance? A: That of a scavenger.

Q: Will you explain the nature of the work that a scavenger has to do? A: The scavenger has to take the brush and sweep under the wheels, and to be under the direction of the spinners and the piecers generally. I frequently had to be under the wheels, and in consequence of the perpetual motion of the machinery, I was liable to accidents constantly. I was very frequently obliged to lie flat, to avoid being run over or caught.

Q: How long did you continue at that employment? A: From a year and a half to two years.

Q: What did you go to then? A: To be a piecer.

Q: Did the employment require you to be upon your feet perpetually? A: It did.

Q: You continued at that employment for how long? A: I was a piecer till I was about 15 or 16 years of age.

Q: What were your hours of labour? A: Fourteen; in some cases, 15 and 16 hours a day.

Q: How had you to be kept up to it? A: During the latter part of the day, I was severely beaten very frequently.

Q: Will you state the effect that the degree of labour had upon your health?

A: I never had good health after I went to the factory. At six years of age I was ruddy and strong; I had not been in the mill long before my colour disappeared, and a state of debility came over me, and a wanness in my appearance.

www.powerinthelandscape.co.uk (accessed 3 May 2013)

This description of working conditions for children in the textile industry is typical of the early nineteenth century. In 1800, there were at least 20 000 apprentices working in the cotton mills, of whom a fifth were under the age of 13 years old. Employment of children had been common practice before the Industrial Revolution, but demand for cheap labour increased with the growth of industry. To satisfy this need, orphans in workhouses throughout the country (particularly from London) were sent to places like the Lancashire cotton mills to work long hours in inhospitable conditions. Additionally, it was common for working-class parents to send their children to work quite willingly from at least the age of 8 years as chimney sweeps or in factories and mines. There were several reasons for this.

In the early decades of the nineteenth century, Britain was experiencing significant economic hardship due to a long war with the French that ended in 1815. Consequently, wages were low and taxes high, so, in poor and labouring families, children became a significant contributor to the household economy. There was little concern about school attendance among the children of such households, because education was not universally regarded as beneficial (on the grounds that it might raise children's expectations beyond their station in life); schooling was not made compulsory until the late nineteenth century. Further, the Christian evangelical view, which was socially well established, represented children as tainted by original sin and having an innately corrupt and evil nature. Work was considered a convenient vehicle to instil discipline and moral values. This attitude starkly contrasts with contemporary views of childhood, which were foreshadowed by the Enlightenment philosopher Jean-Jacques Rousseau (1712–78). He advocated childhood as a precious time, arguing that if children were treated well and educated appropriately, they would grow to become responsible adults and valuable to society: 'Nature wants children to be children before they are men' (*Émile, ou De l'éducation* [Emile, or On Education], 1762).

Discussion point: Contemporary society's reaction to the working conditions of children in the nineteenth century is condemnatory of their exploitation and neglect. Yet the practice of sending children to work from a young age was, to the majority, acceptable. The boundaries between what is and is not acceptable are historically fluid and culturally determined. Thus societies in the future may criticise us for forcing children with little academic ability to attend school until 18 years of age and for putting enormous pressure on children to succeed leading to poor self-esteem and, coupled with other factors, outbreaks of self harm.

Attitudes did slowly alter and eventually children's working conditions improved and their hours of work reduced. There were several drivers of change. The first was the work of a number of philanthropic men, some of whom would have been influenced by Rousseau's ideas regarding the importance of environment to a child's moral as well as physical development. One of the first of these was Jonas Hanway (1712–86). In the 1770s, he tried unsuccessfully to prevent children working as chimney sweeps before the age of 9 years. Another was the Welsh cotton-mill owner and social reformer Robert Owen (1771–1858), who established a model community at New Lanark where crèches were available for working mothers and education was supplied for children and adults. It was he who drove the Cotton Mills and Factory Act 1819, which prohibited children younger than 9 years old from working.

Arguably the most well-known social reformer of the nineteenth century was Lord Anthony Alfred-Cooper Shaftesbury (1801–85), who was dubbed by the working class the Poor Man's Earl. He was responsible for the Factories Act 1833, which applied to children in the cotton mills and factories. This required children between the ages of 9 and 13 years to have 2 hours of education daily, 6 days per week, and their working hours to be reduced. He campaigned for years to improve the lot of chimney sweeps and achieved this with the Chimney Sweepers Act 1875, which, for the first time, provided for police enforcement and brought in licensing of sweeps. This success was partly attributable to the tragic case of George Brewster, a 12-year-old boy illegally apprenticed who was sent up a flue 12 inches by 6 inches at Fulbourn Hospital. He died of lung congestion soon after being dragged out. His master, William Wyer, was convicted for manslaughter and sentenced to hard labour for 6 months. Shaftesbury used the publicity over this case to promote his bill.

Popular fiction also played its role in swinging public opinion. *The Water-Babies, A Fairy Tale for a Land Baby* (1863) was written by Charles Kingsley, a priest, historian and social reformer who, with others, established the Christian socialist movement. The book, which is about the plight of a young chimney sweep who runs away from his employer, became very popular and raised public awareness of the conditions in which sweeps worked. So, too, did Charles Dickens' book *Oliver Twist* (1838), in which the eponymous character is at one point almost apprenticed to Gamfield, a chimney sweep master with the reputation for causing the death of several of his apprentices. Fanny Trollope's novel *Michael Armstrong: factory boy* (1840) was concerned with textile manufacturers and was initially accused by reviewers of having revolutionary potential. A later book, *The Cry of Children from the Brickyards of England: a statement and appeal, with remedy* (1871), by George Smith, described the piteous conditions of children working in this industry; in the same year, an extended Factory and Workshop Act was passed that almost halved the number of under 15-year-olds working in brickyards.

The third driver of change was the public health movement. Two years after Edwin Chadwick's Report on the Sanitary Conditions of the Labouring Poor (1842), the Health of the Towns Association was formed with the aim of firmly establishing the sanitary idea into public policy making and legislation.

The Public Health Act 1848 was subsequently passed, which set up a central department, The General Board of Health, to which local boards of health were accountable. Each local board had to appoint an officer for health whose remit was to identify causes of disease and ways to prevent them. Clearly, the poor working conditions and nutrition of young people and children were to be a concern for these new medical officers.

Whilst there was little appetite for universal elementary education, it was much easier to generate the political will to prepare children for the labour force. The same individuals who campaigned to improve the working conditions of children often also campaigned for children to learn some basic academic skills for deployment at work. Thus, from the outset, many of the Factory Acts required that some time each week be devoted to basic education and religious instruction. Although there was hostility from some quarters to the idea of educating the children of the labouring poor, the number of schools built increased, so that by 1851 most children did attend school although the average duration of attendance was only 2 years. The Elementary Education Act 1870 laid down the principle of universal education for all 5–13-year-olds, but a raft of legislation was needed over the next 20 years to make elementary education free and to render school attendance compulsory with penalties in cases in which children were illegally employed or when parents were resistant to change.

The process of improving the welfare of children was a long and drawn-out affair requiring the redefinition of 'childhood' and a profound change in attitudes. The abuses children experienced were structural, in that they occurred essentially as a result of collective neglect or exploitation leading to poverty, morbidity, premature mortality and educational and social deprivation. To change this required state action and legislation that conferred powers of enforcement.

However, the state was more reluctant to intervene in 'the sacred precinct' of the family home (*see* Section 5, Chapter 1, 'Child safeguarding', for how the child protection movement developed in Britain and the USA).

Why is this relevant?

- In developed countries, we no longer see children forced to earn a living. If they work, it is part-time and of their own volition. This is not the case in poor developing countries where children are still exploited. Just like the nineteenth-century cotton factory owners, we experience the benefits of child labour when we buy cheap clothes from such countries.
- We have created a society in which children and young people are very prone to stress due to the academic demands put on them, including the incessant tests that they must take from the age of 7.
- In 2013, the UK ranked 16th in UNICEF's international league tables of children's overall well-being; data was taken from 29 economically advanced countries. For educational well-being the UK performed particularly poorly, ranked at 24th. www.unicef.org.uk

Further reading

Brockliss L, Montgomery L, editors. *Childhood and Violence in the Western Tradition.* Oxford: Oxbow; 2010.

Kirby P. *Child Labour in Britain, 1750–1870.* Basingstoke and New York, NY: Palgrave Macmillan; 2003.

National Archives. *Human Rights.* Available at: www.nationalarchives.gov.uk/humanrights (accessed 5 January 2013).

Piper C. Moral campaigns for children's welfare in the nineteenth century. In: Hendrick H, editor. *Child Welfare and Social Policy: an essential reader.* Bristol: Policy Press; 2005. pp. 13–30.

www.parliament.uk. *Living Heritage.* Available at: www.parliament.uk/about/living-heritage (accessed 5 January 2013).

8

Water as a historical force

A PHYSICAL CONSTANT FOR THE HUMAN CONDITION IS THE NEED FOR water. It is a prerequisite for comfort, hydration and function at the level of the body as an organism, and at the cellular level for respiration, digestion and virtually every process, major or minor, necessary to survival. Access to potable water, and pressure on it as a resource, can explain early settlement patterns, the success or failure of military endeavour, the prosperity of industry and the basis of geographical disputes.

Water has also been used for the disposal of waste products through the ages. It is the medium for bathing, either for ritual or cleanliness purposes, and the means of ridding communities of human excreta. Where population densities remain low, people have historically used natural water courses such as rivers to flush away waste. However, the rise of cities globally presented humankind with a watery problem: how to retain supplies of fresh water for drinking or food production without polluting the source.

The first global pandemic of cholera morbus emanated from south-east Asia in the late 1810s and spread to Europe and Russia; it arrived in Britain in 1831. Contemporaries had no accurate ideas about how it was spread or what to do to combat the infection, since germ theory, which explained infectious transmission, was not to be proven until the mid-1860s through Louis Pasteur's (1822–95) experiments (see Section 4, Chapter 4, 'The germ theory of disease'). A Central Board of Health was hastily established to address cholera administratively, but the advice issued by the board could not have had any prophylactic effect. It recommended 'The true Preventatives are a healthy Body, and a cheerful, unruffled Mind' (printed advice from the Central Board of Health in Whitehall, 1831. Derbyshire Record Office D2057A/PO2/372); unfortunately, the condition of most British cities was perfectly tuned for the transmission of cholera to thousands of people, regardless of their state of mind.

The country experienced rapid population growth in the 1810s and 1820s, and economic factors ensured that an increasing proportion of this population sought a living in towns and cities. Flushing toilets were virtually unknown. The very wealthy might have a private earth closet or midden on their property, but most people had access to a shared privy or routinely disposed of sewage in the streets. Moreover, there was a perfect overlap between the source of drinking water and the waterways used to get rid of dirty water. In Birmingham, for example, the River Tame was black with sewage in the 1850s but remained the city's main source of water.

> **Question**: John Snow (1813–58) first disseminated his theory that cholera was waterborne in 1849. How did *The Lancet* and other medical journals react to his idea?

Cholera infected people of all social classes but was most prevalent among the poor and ordinary working people. Historian Margaret Pelling has argued that this social distinction among victims delayed an effective official response to cholera: those in power were not the most likely to suffer. Public health legislation eventually attempted to address the overcrowding, squalor and insanitary conditions of Britain's cities. It is likely, though, that quarantine at British ports and other measures were equally responsible, or more responsible, for ensuring that cholera did not reach epidemic proportions in any year after 1866.

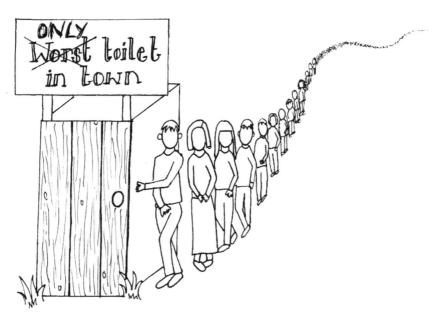

Rendering houses habitable in the modern sense of supplying clean piped water and access to toilets connected to sewers took much longer to achieve. Domestic water supplies had become cleaner, continuous and commonly available by the 1890s, but it was generally easier to demolish houses and build afresh than to connect existing properties to sewers. As a result, well into the twentieth century, large swathes of urban populations had to use shared middens that were unconnected to sewers.

Why is this relevant?

- Shock epidemics, that kill tens, hundreds or thousands of people very quickly, are a feature of overcrowded urbanised life.
- At the time of writing, the world is experiencing its seventh global pandemic of cholera. While we now have a much better understanding of how it is spread, financial imperatives still govern access to both clean water and effective treatment. It is still the world's poorest citizens who are most likely to contract and die from cholera.
- Medical research that contradicts a prevailing orthodoxy can take a long time to become generally accepted or to overturn preferred theories. This remains the case, despite the advance of scientific method and knowledge.

Further reading

Pelling M. *Cholera, Fever and English Medicine, 1825–1865.* Oxford: Oxford University Press; 1978.

Smith FB. *The People's Health, 1830–1910.* London: Croom Helm; 1979.

Wohl AS. *Endangered Lives: public health in Victorian Britain.* London: Methuen; 1984.

Section 5

The challenges of life: childhood, disability, ageing and mental illness

1

Child safeguarding

My father and mother are both dead. I don't know how old I am. I have no recollection of a time when I did not live with the Connollys ... Mamma has been in the habit of whipping and beating me almost every day ... I have now the black and blue marks on my head ... and also a cut on the left side of my forehead which was made by a pair of scissors ... I have no recollection of ever having been kissed by any one ... I never dared to speak to anybody, because if I did I would get whipped ... I do not know for what I was whipped – mamma never said anything to me when she whipped me. I do not want to go back to live with mamma, because she beats me so.

Testimony of Mary Ellen Wilson, 10 April 1874

Watkins SA. The Mary Ellen Myth: correcting child welfare history. *Social Work.* 1990; **35**(6): 500–3.

In nineteenth-century Britain and the USA, there was little state interference in child-rearing practices within the family. It was assumed that the father of the house had a right to do as he pleased. In 1892, one British lawyer argued that the murder of a child by its father was legal, since parents had absolute rights over their children (Jones D. *Understanding Child Abuse.* London: Macmillan Press. 1987. p 43). Mary Ellen Wilson's case was the first child-abuse case to reach the law courts. At that time, there was no child protection law; her advocates had to resort to invoking an animal protection law by arguing that she was a human animal. The following year, animal rights campaigners in New York established the Society for Prevention of Cruelty to Children, which was dedicated to protecting children in their family homes. Similar societies became established across the USA. The movement inspired the creation of the National Society for the Prevention of Cruelty to Children (NSPCC) in Britain, following a visit to the USA from Thomas Agnew, a Liverpool banker, who facilitated the establishment of the first Society for the Prevention of Cruelty to Children in the UK, at Liverpool in 1883.

Although child employment legislation in the USA trailed behind that in Britain, the former continued to take the lead in child welfare systems. Both countries initially favoured institutional care for children who were unable to remain with their families, but adoption and foster care became the preferred option in the USA of the early twentieth century. This was due to the first White House Conference on Children and Youth in 1909 on the subject of care of dependent children. In contrast, Britain did not legalise adoption until 1926 and even then there was no provision for the monitoring or regulation of adoptive families. Institutional care remained the preferred option and was used heavily following the Second World War due to a policy to emigrate poor and orphaned children to Commonwealth countries. Children often found themselves in large isolated institutions in which work regimes were hard, sometimes brutal, and the discipline strict. Latterly, the British Government has acknowledged its mistake in adhering to this policy and apologised.

Child protection faded from the forefront of the political agenda until the early 1960s when the American paediatrician Dr C Henry Kempe and psychiatrist Brandt F Steele published a paper entitled 'The battered child syndrome' in which they explored the prevalence of abuse and its presentation. A year later in 1963 the *British Medical Journal* published a report called *Multiple Epiphseal Injuries in Babies* (Griffiths D. and Moynihan FJ.) containing the new term 'battered child syndrome' and citing Kempe and Steele's paper. The American response was swift, with the passing of the 1962 Social Security Act, which required every state to have minimum standards of child protection legislation; the government now held responsibility for the protection of children across the country. In contrast, in Britain, although the NSPCC undertook significant research into the prevalence and nature of child physical abuse, there had been no legislative change in child protection since The Childrens and Young Persons Act 1933. However, the death of Maria Colwell in 1973, aged 7 years, led to an inquiry the following year that resulted in the government establishing Area Child Protection Committees, responsible for ensuring the safety of children at risk. Nevertheless, over the following years, gaps in the child protection services were revealed by several further child deaths. In 1989, two years following the Cleveland report (Butler-Sloss E. *Report of the Inquiry into Child Abuse in Cleveland*) the Children Act was passed which permitted intervention if a child was suffering from harm and asserted the rights of children to protection from abuse and exploitation; however, the main aim of this legislation was to support families more effectively so that children were not prematurely removed from their home. In this same year, the United Nations Convention on the Rights of the Child was opened for signatures. This remains the most complete statement of children's rights ever produced and the most widely ratified international human rights treaty in history. Significantly, the treaty is very child-centric in that it not only prioritises the best interests of the child but respects the child's views; for example, Article 12 of the convention explicates 'every child has a right . . . to have their views taken seriously'.

It may seem anomalous that one of the two countries that has not ratified the United Nations treaty is the USA, given that in 1912 President William Taft set up the United States Children's Bureau, the first national government office in the world with a remit to focus on the well-being of children and their mothers.

The bureau was also tasked with researching, evaluating and recommending policy reform. Over the years, it has provided evidence-based data to the media and political campaigns to support legislative change. In Britain, the Home Office Children's Department never had the advantage of a research unit and most reform has come about through the recommendations resulting from reactive inquiries. Possibly the most significant inquiry since the death of Maria Colwell occurred following Victoria Climbié's death in 2000. Lord William Laming's *The Victoria Climbié Inquiry: report of 2003*, which highlighted numerous missed opportunities to intervene, made several recommendations that included establishing a minister for children, a national agency for children and families, a national child database and a 24-hour helpline for the public to report concerns about children. In 2009, following the death of 'Baby P', Laming produced *The Protection of Children in England: a progress report*, which criticised local authorities for failing to implement his 2003 recommendations. In 2011, another government-commissioned report, *The Munro Review of Child Protection: final report – a child-centred system* reported on an inquiry led by Professor Eileen Munro and led to further changes in child-safeguarding arrangements in the UK.

Why is this relevant?

- Although the current efficacy of British and American approaches to child protection is probably similar, the approaches are very different. The British system is more reactive and dependent on the recommendations of inquiries. The American system is possibly more suited to identifying systemic flaws earlier, thanks to having a well-established central board with a research and evaluative remit.
- The UN Convention on the Rights of the Child suffers from the same difficulties that legislation did in Britain for most of the nineteenth century. It has set out laudable principles but will be unable to establish them worldwide until they become enforceable.

Further reading

Dow C, Phillips J. *'Forgotten Australians' and 'Lost Innocents': child migrants and children in institutional care in Australia* [background note]. Canberra: Parliamentary Library; 2009. Available at: www.aph.gov.au/binaries/library/pubs/bn/sp/childmigrants.pdf (accessed 19 April 2013).

Hendrick H. *Child Welfare: England 1872–1989*. New York, NY: Routledge; 1994.

Jalongo M. The story of Mary Ellen Wilson: tracing the origins of child protection in America. *Early Childhood Educational Journal*. 2006; **34**(1): 1–4.

Pragnall C. *The Cleveland Sexual Abuse Scandal: an abuse and misuse of professional power*. Available at: www.davidlane.org/children/choct2002/choct2002/pragnell%20cleveland%20abuse.html (accessed 15 December 2012).

2

Two steps forward,
one step back: disability

ACCORDING TO AN ARTICLE ENTITLED 'PARALYMPICS 2012: THE ELLIE Simmonds' legend continues to grow with bronze to add to her collection' (P Hayward, *The Telegraph*, 5 September 2012), Ellie Simmonds, who has achondroplasia, read the 2005 teenage novel *Uglies*, by Scott Westerfeld, while waiting to compete in her events. The book is a science fiction novel set in a future world where, on reaching 16 years, everyone undergoes cosmetic surgery to make them beautiful. This seems somewhat ironic given the popularity of the 2012 Paralympics, which suggests that contemporary societies throughout the world fully accept and indeed celebrate diversity and 'imperfection'.

The present and past attitudes of a society to disability can be illuminated by the legislation passed by that society. The first legislation in England that acknowledged the needs of the disabled was the Statute of Cambridge 1388. This divided the poor into 'deserving' and 'undeserving' and allowed the former, which included the disabled and older people, to claim alms. The Poor Relief Act 1601 required each parish to support the deserving poor, thereby initiating general taxation to achieve this; however, to ask for support and qualify for alms, an applicant had to assume the role of grateful and apologetic supplicant. Today, some would argue that nothing has fundamentally changed, given that the conditions that must be met to receive disability living benefits in Britain can be arduous and, further, that a failure to conform to the way the government believes disabled people should behave leads to hardship and often significant emotional distress.

Question 1: What benefits are available to those with disability in England and Wales?

Historically, societal reaction to disability has ranged from fear and ostracism to attempts at integration and, latterly, acknowledgement of the value of all people to the community. The legend of the 'changeling', which exists in several cultures, perhaps best exemplifies the stigma of having a baby that seems disabled or at least different to the norm. Given this situation, parents preferred to believe that their child had been replaced by the offspring of legendary creatures such as trolls, fairies or elves. William Shakespeare's *A Midsummer Night's Dream* alludes to this belief, with Titania and Oberon fighting over possession of a human boy.

Further, the notion that disability was a punishment is embedded in Judeo-Christian religion. For example, in the Old Testament it is stated in Deuteronomy that 'if humans are immoral they will be blinded by God' and in Matthew in the New Testament there is a description of Jesus curing a man with palsy after saying his sins are forgiven. St Augustine considered impairment a 'punishment for the fall of Adam and other sins' and Martin Luther saw the devil in a disabled child and recommended its death. Indeed, infanticide was advocated in the ancient world for the sickly and weak, for they were considered of little economic worth and a burden to their parents. Thus, the Greek physician Soranus of Ephesus in the second century AD advises on how to recognise a child worth raising. Some of those who were not killed would be destined to be a source of entertainment in the Roman games, in which, for example, dwarfs and blind men were put to fight animals and women. The clever but deformed Emperor Claudius was almost put to death at birth. He was subsequently dismissed by his mother as 'a monster: a man whom Nature had begun to work upon and flung aside' (Suetonius. *The Twelve Caesars*. London: Penguin Classics; 2007. p. 180). Putting children and adults with physical abnormalities on display for amusement and profit was embodied in the 'freak shows' of the Victorian age in England, such as at Bartholomew Fair in Smithfield, London, where the public could see Siamese twins, dwarfs and giants. A similar process of display and ridicule occurred in Bethlem, the first hospital for the mentally ill in England, until the doors were closed to the public in 1770. Arguably, television shows like *So You Think You Can Dance* (2009) also parade the disabled for amusement. However, these examples of how the disabled have been treated in a degrading way across time are eclipsed by the Nazi Aktion [action] T4 euthanasia programme of the Second World War.

Question 2: What was the aim of Aktion T4 in 1939?

Segregation into institutions was a common response to the disabled, particularly during the British industrial era. An example of this was the behaviour of charitable organisations for the blind in the nineteenth century. These would recruit young blind men to learn a trade but discourage fraternisation with the sighted community; strict discipline and religious observance were expected. Being separated from the sighted community could lead to isolation and loss of previous natural support networks. Pay was low and educational standards worse than in state schools. For a long time, it was felt that the blind did not need to learn to read, so Braille was not introduced in Britain until the 1880s, whereas it had been officially endorsed in France in 1853. Finding employment in the sighted community after leaving their institution was difficult without any provision for aftercare. In 1899 the National League of the Blind was established through the aggregation of several blind societies, blind clubs and workshops. Its main aim was to campaign for legislation to secure for blind people the right to work, state funding for training and employment on a 'living wage'; and pensions, rather than poor relief, for those blind people unable to work.

In 1920, the Blind Persons Act allowed the blind to claim entitlements such as pensions. To implement this required an objective definition of blindness, but the only definition at this time was that of 'economic' blindness, namely, an inability to perform work for which eyesight was essential. Thirteen years later, the Snellen test was introduced as a standard test for certifying blindness. An unexpected outcome was that the number on the blind register able to claim a pension increased, because the test identified those who had been previously found as having merely bad or failing eyesight.

Question 3: What is the Snellen test?

In 1948, the Labour Government passed the National Assistance Act. By then, the prevailing ideology had changed. The disabled were no longer to be segregated but mainstreamed. The numbers of specialist schools and workshops were reduced and employment alongside the 'able' was encouraged. In William Henry Beveridge's new welfare state, the aim was to enable the disabled to live as normal a life as possible within the larger community; however, personal social services remained subject to administrative assessment by local government officers, who, together with other professionals, tended to decide what the disabled needed. This was addressed somewhat by the 1996 Community Care (Direct Payments) Act, which brought in a policy of personalisation of care. The disabled could now determine what care they received and from whom rather than this being determined by someone else.

Many government policies have been criticised by the UK's disability movement for identifying the individual as the problem rather than viewing disability as a social construct. The movement argues that, given universal access, a person in a wheelchair is no longer disabled. A good example of validity of the concept of disability being a social construct can be seen in a community who lived in Martha's Vineyard, an island off the Massachusetts coast, in the nineteenth century. In that community, a gene for deafness was highly prevalent: 1 in 155 people were deaf here by the turn of the century compared with 1 in 6000 on the mainland. The community responded by creating its own sign language, which was used by all the inhabitants, deaf or not. A major criticism of the medical model of health and ill-health is that it portrays the individual as the one with a problem that should be medically corrected if possible, rather than society being at fault for having a low tolerance of difference.

Why is this relevant?

- The disabled community has endured a consistent history of being stigmatised by being ignored, segregated, laughed at, humiliated and researched. They have also been victims of the eugenics movement. It is debatable whether this stigma will ever disappear.

- Definitions of disability change, as shown with the Snellen test for blindness. In the future, could genetic technology widen the definition of disability to embrace people with some 'unwanted' genes?
- Debates about who should qualify for state support have been played out for centuries.
- Everyone has the potential to be disabled through accident, illness or old age; it is part of the human condition. Perhaps society should perceive 'disability' as a fluid condition into which any one of us may drop temporarily or permanently.

Further reading

Borsay A. *Disability and Social Policy in Britain since 1750: a history of exclusion.* Basingstoke: Palgrave Macmillan; 2009.

3

Broken bones and failing joints

FRACTURES AND ARTHRITIS HAVE ALWAYS BEEN BOTH A FEATURE OF human life and conditions that attracted intervention. Neolithic skeletal remains suggest that the technique of splinting was used to treat fractures even then. Arthritic conditions have been identified in bones found in Egyptian burial sites dated to about 3000 BC. Descriptions of arthritis and a treatment for a broken upper arm are found in the *Edwin Smith Papyrus*, an Ancient Egyptian text that has been dated to 2000 BC. In about the fifth century BC, Hippocrates (c. 460–c. 370 BC) wrote a *Treatise on Fractures and Dislocations*, in which he addressed the subjects of compound fractures, reduction and dressings. Many of his sound principles of management are followed today. One such recommendation was that of early mobilisation of fractures once reduced: 'It should be kept in mind that exercise strengthens and inactivity wastes'. He also described arthritis, observing that it affected mainly the young when it was associated with fever. His aphorisms on the subject of gout, which he distinguished from other joint conditions, include:

- 'Eunachs do not take the gout, nor become bald'
- 'A youth does not get gout before sexual intercourse'
- 'A woman does not take the gout unless her menses be stopped'
- 'In gouty affections, inflammation subsides within 40 days'
- 'Gouty afflictions become active in spring and autumn'

Hippocrates. Aphorisms. Section VI.

Question: Would you agree with these statements?

Spinal deformity was very common in the seventeenth and eighteenth centuries and was often due to rickets or scrofula (*see* Section 4, Chapter 1, 'The "King's Evil" or "wasting disease": tuberculosis'). In 1601, the Poor Relief Act was passed in England; this was the first legislation in England to consider the plight of the 'crippled' and provide for them. Hitherto, the 'deformed and lame' were ostracised, partly because of the belief that their disability was a punishment from God (*see* the previous chapter, 'Two steps forward, one step back: disability').

From the Middle Ages to the early nineteenth century, the old skill of bone setting was the preserve of carpenters, blacksmiths and retired sailors. One exception was Sally Map, a female bone setter who was paid by the town of Epsom in 1736 to reside there to set bones. Gradually, medical men acquired this skill and bone setters disappeared as the new speciality of orthopaedics developed, although its clear distinction from other branches of medicine only occurred during the First World War. The term 'orthopaedics' was coined by the French physician Nicholas Andry (1658–1742) in a paper called *L'orthopedie*, published in 1741 and translated into English two years later (*Treatise on Preventing Diseases in Children*); the Greek word *orthos*, means straight – that is, free from deformity – and *paidios* means child. An interest in childhood deformities is a theme that runs through the early history of the speciality. For example, Jacques Delpech (1777–1832) was the first surgeon to attempt to treat the condition of club foot in 1816. Georg Friedrich Louis Stromeyer (1804–76) continued Delpech's work and, in 1831, successfully operated on a 14-year-old boy at his hospital, which was to become a centre for the study of deformities and their treatment. An English surgeon, William John Little (1810–94), visited Stromeyer's hospital and had his own deformed foot, the result of childhood poliomyelitis, successfully operated on by him. He returned to England, where he taught the 'Stromeyer technique' at his hospital, which became the Royal Orthopaedic Hospital in 1843. Another example is that of Robert Jones (1857–1933), who, together with Agnes Hunt, established a hospital for crippled children in Baschurch in 1904. Jones was the nephew of Welsh surgeon Hugh Thomas (1834–91), who invented the Thomas splint, an iron leg with a ring at one end to facilitate extension of the injured limb. He had done pioneering work on fractures and deformities and also advocated 'carrying through treatment'. By this he meant that a skilled orthopaedist should oversee recovery once a fracture had been joined to ensure that the union remained optimal. Many decades later, he was proved correct by a follow-up study on 3000 fractures reduced by relatively inexperienced doctors, the findings of which were published in the *British Medical Journal* in 1912 (*Report of the Fractures Committee*). The outcomes were extremely poor.

Jones did much to publicise his uncle's work but is remembered in his own right for establishing first-aid posts to quickly handle injuries sustained by any of the 20 000 workers on the Manchester ship canal project, a 36-mile canal linking Manchester and Liverpool. His extensive experience in the late 1880s of managing fractures whilst Surgeon-Superintendent for the project led the army to ask him to organise rehabilitation of the wounded in the First World War.

The first complete description of rheumatoid arthritis was written in 1800 by Augustin Jacob Landré-Beauvais (1772–1840). A separate condition associated with fever as well as painful and swollen joints had been well described by another French physician, Guillaume de Baillou (1538–1616), as well as by Thomas Sydenham (1624–89), the 'English Hippocrates', who had also tried to differentiate gout, febrile and non-febrile rheumatism. Sydenham gave an accurate description for the febrile condition (what we now know to be rheumatic fever), noting that it tended to occur in the young and vigorous, and that it began with chills and fever followed by a polyarthritis. It is not clear whether Sydenham saw this as a distinct disease and different to chronic non-febrile rheumatism (now known as osteoarthritis or rheumatoid arthritis) or took it to be a variation of chronic rheumatism. In the 1870s, uncertainty continued about whether rheumatic fever and rheumatoid arthritis were distinctly different diseases. Between 1885 and 1895, the possibility of a bacterial aetiology for both presentations began to be entertained, but it was not until the 1940s that a bacterial cause was demonstrated for rheumatic fever and disproven for rheumatoid arthritis.

Without any real understanding of the aetiology of either acute or chronic rheumatism, it is not surprising that to contemporary eyes past treatments may seem random. Many interventions were influenced by humoral theory or based on folklore; some were palliative. Fever was dealt with by bleeding and treating pain: 'when considerable, half a grain of opium may be added to three grains of antimonial powder . . . to be taken every four or six hours' (R Thomas, *A Treatise on Domestic Medicine*, 1822). The same book advises on 'proper evacuation' of the bowels, 'flannel cloths wrung out in warm water' for affected joints and, on remission, Peruvian bark. In England, taking the waters at spas such as Bath or Buxton was recommended for chronic rheumatism, 'but bathing in these waters is only proper where the disease is unaccompanied by inflammation and in which the pains are not increased by warmth when the patient is in bed'. Thomas further suggests that in obstinate cases that do not respond to the above measures, caustic soda should be applied to the joint 'together with electricity or galvinism'. As far back as in 1763, the Reverend Edmund Stone had discovered that willow bark was helpful, but this discovery was not scientifically proven until a Scottish doctor, Thomas John MacLagan published a paper in 1876, The willow as a remedy for acute rheumatism, in the *Lancet*. However, the process of extraction and separation to a pure state was costly and the side effects of salicyclic acid proved troublesome; it took almost another 30 years to find a way of commercially manufacturing aspirin and over a century for the beneficial effects of steroids to be discovered.

Gout was seen as a disease of the wealthy. 'Be temperate in wine, in eating, girls, and cloth, or the Gout will seize you and plague you both', wrote Benjamin Franklin in a *Dialogue between Franklin and Gout* in 1780 (www.gutenberg.org [accessed 14 May 2013]); he enjoyed all these pleasures and was indeed afflicted with the gout for many years. In 1900, *The Times* declared '[t]he common cold is well named, but the gout seems instantly to raise the patient's status'.

Although hereditary factors were recognised as contributory to the condition, the main cause was the upper-class habit of drinking sweet and fortified wines and eating a diet rich in starch and protein. The idea that overindulgence, including in sexual activities, was the culprit seems to go back to Hippocrates' time. Writing some centuries later, the Roman Stoic philosopher Seneca (4 BC–65 AD) wryly observed that although gout was a disease mostly of males, 'in this age women rival men in every kind of lasciviousness . . . why need we be surprised at seeing so many of the female sex with gout' (c. 54–65 AD).(archive.org/stream/goutoollew.)

Robert Thomas writes in *A Treatise on Domestic Medicine* that the causes include 'too free indulgence in the use of animal food, fermented liquors, and venery, leading a sedentary and studious life, [and] anxiety of mind'. Not surprisingly, he recommended that 'strict temperance' should be the mainstay of treatment.

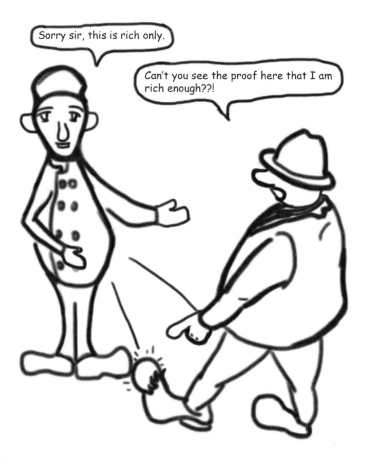

Humoral theory explained that gout was due to an excessive amount of humour dropping into a joint. Thus, the name *gutta*, a Latin word meaning 'drop', although in Classical times the name varied according to location: 'podagra' if afflicting the big toe, 'gonagra' for the knee and 'chiagra' for the hands. It was an English physician, Alfred Garrod (1819–1907), who identified uric acid crystals in gout tophi and devised a bedside test to differentiate gout from rheumatoid arthritis in 1848 – the thread test. His *A Treatise on Gout and Rheumatic Gout (Rheumatoid Arthritis)* of 1876 suggested that reducing purine-rich food could help to control the disease. The structure and synthesis of the purine protein was discovered by a German chemist, Hermann Emil Fischer (1852–1919), for which he won the Nobel Prize in Medicine in 1902.

The earliest pharmacological intervention for gout was that of colchicine, which comes from the bulb of autumn crocus. This is mentioned in the *Ebers*

Papyrus (c. 1550 BC). Alexander de Tralles administered it for acute gout in the sixth century AD and it was still being recommended by the French surgeon Ambrose Pare (1510–94) a thousand years later; however, its severe gastrointestinal side effects limited its use. Allopurinol, which reduces the production of uric acid, was produced by George H Hitchings (1905–98) and Gertrude Belle Elion (1918–99) who won the Nobel Prize in Medicine in 1988 for its discovery.

Why is this relevant?

- Whereas understanding the causes of conditions affecting the joints did not occur until the late nineteenth and early twentieth centuries, risk factors and symptomatic treatments were identified over two millennia ago in Ancient Greece due to good clinical observation and the experiential nature of Hippocratic medical practice (*see* Section 6, Chapter 1, 'Early Greek and Roman contributions').
- Acquiring the skill to manage fractures was a very early human achievement, probably because a broken limb bone presents an obvious physical problem with a relatively simple non-invasive solution.

Further reading

Beckett D. From bonesetters to orthopaedic surgeons: a history of the specialty of orthopaedics. *The Surgical Technologist*. 1999; November: 7–19. Available at: www.ast.org/pdf/Professionals/Ortho_CE_Package_Consolidated.pdf (accessed 19 April 2013).

Thomas R. *The Way to Preserve Good Health Together with A Treatise on Domestic Medicine*. London: T and G Underwood; 1822.

Hart FD. History of the treatment of rheumatoid arthritis. *British Medical Journal*. 1976; 1(6012): 763–5.

Ponseti IV. History of orthopaedic surgery. *Iowa Orthopedic Journal*. 1991; 11: 59–64.

4

Ageing and the good death

[M]y old age sits light upon me ..., and not only is not burdensome, but is even happy. For as Nature has marked the bounds of everything else, so she has marked the bounds of life. Moreover, old age is the final scene, as it were, in life's drama, from which we ought to escape when it grows wearisome and, certainly, when we have had our fill.

Cicero, *De Senectute* [On old age], 44 BC

THE DEFINITION OF 'OLD AGE' AND THE SIGNIFICANCE OR MEANING of older life have varied according to epoch and culture. The Ancient Greeks indicated four life stages: childhood, youth, maturity and old age, which would seem quite modern but for the belief that the characteristics of each stage were determined by the humours, qualities, elements and seasons. Aristotle (384–322 BC) divided life into three stages: growth, stasis and decline; the last was a time when normal failings became magnified, passions waned and the loss of the body's innate heat depressed the spirit. The Ptolemaic version (c. second century BC) held that there were seven stages, which reflected the divine order of the universe. The sixth stage was ruled by Jupiter and occurred from the age of 56 to 68 years; this was a time of thoughtfulness, dignity and decorum. But by the final stage, ruled by Saturn, people became dispirited, weak, hard to please and easily offended. This version of life's stages lasted well into the Middle Ages and is revisited in William Shakespeare's famous 'seven ages of man' monologue, spoken by a dispirited Jaques in Act 2, Scene 7 of *As You like it*. Galen (129–c. 200 AD) also adopted a humoral and pessimistic view: 'For that which all men commonly call old age is the dry and cold constitution of the body resulting from many years of life.' (*On Youth and Old Age*) Although he did not consider old age to be a disease, neither was it a fully healthy time. His suggestions for amelioration included reading aloud, ball throwing and travel in ships; perhaps this is why cruises are so popular with the contemporary older person! In contrast, the philosopher, statesman and senator, Cicero (106–43 BC) had a more sanguine attitude:

[E]njoy the blessing of strength while you have it and do not bewail it when it is gone unless ... you believe that youth must lament the loss of infancy, or

> early manhood the passing of youth. Life's race-course is fixed; Nature has only a single path and that path is run but once, and to each stage of existence has been allotted its own appropriate quality; so that the weakness of childhood, the impetuosity of youth, the seriousness of middle life, the maturity of old age – each bears some of Nature's fruit, which must be garnered in its own season.
>
> *De Senectute* [On Old Age]

Perhaps he therefore did not mind too much when he was assassinated at the age of 63.

Not much was written about female old age, although the menopause was the subject of Graeco-Roman drama in which women were mocked with allusions to their ability to 'wither fruit on the vine' or 'crack a mirror' (*see* Section 3, Chapter 7, 'The "change": menopause and its meanings'). A Medieval text, *De Secretis Mulierum* [Women's secrets], reflected the orthodox humoral paradigm of disease in which cessation of menses implied that menstrual fluid was retained inside the body, giving rise to toxic vapours. The menopause tends to occur sometime between 45 and 55 years of age, whereas the common definition of 'old age' from antiquity to the eighteenth century was older than this. It would therefore appear that women were deemed elderly and, indeed, somewhat repulsive at an earlier age than men.

Contrary to modern preconceptions, the biblical ideal of living to be three score and 10 years old was not that unusual to achieve. Although life expectancy at birth in the seventeenth century was far lower than it is today, this was chiefly determined by loss of life in infancy and early childhood. A further common misconception is that older people were always supported by their families. Many older people who were poor had no children, partly because of the high infant mortality rate but also because even if their children did survive, they sometimes either were too poor to help their parents or had emigrated. In the seventeenth century, about one-third of women had no surviving children.

Question 1: What happened to older people who were poor before the twentieth century?

Social and medical approaches to the dying have also varied according to era. Following the devastation wrought by the Black Death in the fourteenth century, the Catholic Church commissioned a text called *Ars moriendi* [The art of dying], which offered advice on how to prepare for death. A shorter version consisted of 11 pictures that communicated the main points to the illiterate. A person's main concern then was to save his or her soul and to put domestic and financial matters in order. Seeking forgiveness and preparing to meet one's God continued to be the dominant narrative of a good death until more secular times. The medical profession did not take much of a role in the care of the dying and indeed was criticised in the nineteenth century for being more interested in cure than care. Thus, a number of hospices were established by Christian organisations to care for this group of patients in whom medical practitioners had little interest. One physician who was interested in the dying process was William Munk (1816–98). Munk wrote a book called *Euthanasia: or, medical treatment in aid of an easy death* (1887), which espoused a holistic and humane approach advocating simple measures to relieve discomfort, avoidance of treatment that prolonged the dying process and, most importantly, sufficient opium for pain relief. It was enthusiastically received by nurses and medical practitioners.

The following event perhaps signposted a new and different interpretation of euthanasia:

> In the early hours of 12 November 1915, at Chicago's German-American Hospital, Anna Bollinger gave birth to her fourth child, a seven-pound baby boy...the baby was blue and badly deformed. After conferring with the father, the doctor awakened Harry J. Haiselden, the hospital's forty-five-year-old chief of staff. Haiselden diagnosed a litany of physical defects...He predicted that, without surgery...the child would die shortly...

Five days later the infant died; Dr Haiselden and the parents had decided not to perform any surgery. This case caused significant interest among the American public and stimulated debate about the moral issues of euthanasia. By the 1930s, a survey showed that 45% of Americans said that they thought that 'mercy killing of infants born permanently deformed or mentally handicapped' was acceptable. In 1938, the first society for euthanasia was established in the USA, which came to be known as the Euthanasia Society of America (ESA); a Voluntary Euthanasia Society (VES) in England had already been founded in 1935 by a retired public health doctor, C. Killick Millard. Both these societies embraced a definition of euthanasia that included termination of life when appealed for by the patient. The next 20 years saw increasing dissatisfaction with the medical management of death. A British Army doctor, Hugh Llewellyn Glyn-Hughes conducted a survey in 1957 that highlighted the lack of provision of services for the dying. One example given was that, in 1956, the majority of people (60%) who died were left to do so at home. Dr Glyn-Hughes who was prominent in founding the Royal College of General Practitioners, was particularly critical of doctors' training, which did not equip them with the skills to provide appropriate physical and psychological care to the terminally ill. It was in this context that Cicely Saunders (1918–2005) pioneered the hospice movement with its emphasis on multidisciplinary holistic care.

Question 2: What changes have since occurred that may have improved the care of older people and the dying?

The number of people who died in hospital in the UK increased from 40% in 1956 to almost 80% by 2010. However, public preference has swung to a wish to die at home. A British strategy to enable people to do so, the National End of Life Care Strategy (2008), seems to have made some inroads into reversing institutionalised dying.

The search for immortality or eternal youth has a long history that has persisted until today, as attested by the following, rather far-fetched-sounding, project:

> **Russian research project offers 'immortality' to billionaires – by transplanting their brains into robot bodies**
> - Contacted list of world's richest to offer immortality
> - Will personally oversee brain transplant into robot body
> - Entrepreneur claims to have 30 scientists working on project
> - Aims to 'transplant' human mind into robot body in 10 years
> - Claims 'next stage' of science is to create a 'new human body'
> - 'This project is leading to immortality,' says Dmitry Itskov
>
> R Waugh, *MailOnline*, 18 July 2012

Anti-ageing measures have always been popular – from Galen, who advocated the 'non-naturals' (good air, diet, sleep, exercise, mental health), to Paracelsus' quest for the philosopher's stone, which was thought to rejuvenate and possibly impart immortality. This interest has been reflected in the popular literature across the centuries – for example, as in Jonathan Swift's *Gulliver's Travels* (1726), which describes the protagonist's travels to imaginary countries, including a place where older immortals live, the struldbrugs. Other examples include *The Picture of Dorian Gray* (1890) by Oscar Wilde, in which the handsome young Dorian never ages, and, more recently, *The Hitchhiker's Guide to the Galaxy* (1979) by Douglas Adams. Probably as much quackery occurs now as in the past: while there used to be sales of Mrs Winslow's soothing syrup, which unbeknown to consumers contained morphine, there are now anti-wrinkle creams and collagen drinks.

Why is this relevant?

- The treatment of marginalised and vulnerable sectors of the population has historically varied. Those who are dying constitute a particularly vulnerable group. Responses are dependent on the interplay of prevailing social, cultural, medical and economic factors.
- Capitalist societies put particular emphasis on productivity. This puts the non-productive at risk of loss of status and decreasing standards of care. This was particularly the case during the Great Depression of the 1930s. Since 2007, social and healthcare funding in the budgets of first-world nations has been significantly reduced owing to global economic instability. This has caused significant hardship for diverse and vulnerable social groups across the world.
- As medical science advances, there is a growing possibility of not only prolonging life further but also of achieving immortality. The human species will have to address the ethical and legal challenges of these possibilities.
- There is still significant controversy about both how the dying are treated and the subject of euthanasia.

Further reading

Thane P, editor. *The Long History of Old Age.* London: Thames and Hudson; 2005.

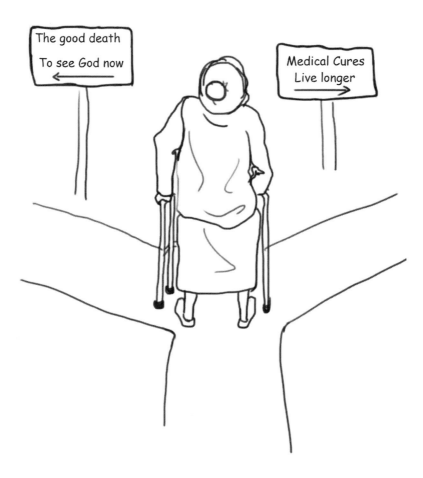

5

What price immortality?

MORTALITY IS AN INHERENT ASPECT OF THE HUMAN CONDITION BUT some parts of individual people can have a much longer 'life' as anatomical preparations or specimens. Specimens for teaching or research purposes have been collected in significant numbers since the late eighteenth century, when clear glass containers and clear alcohol both became technically possible and relatively inexpensive. In the late twentieth and early twenty-first centuries, organ gathering and retention are activities subject to strict rules, particularly surrounding the informed consent of individuals or families concerning the disposal of bodies.

The most skilled and avid collector of specimens in the late eighteenth century was probably John Hunter (1728–93), the leading anatomist and inspiring teacher. He enthusiastically dissected human and animal corpses and became financially indebted in order to acquire unusual material. However, he was notably unscrupulous; for example, he acquired the cadaver of an Irishman, Charles O'Byrne (or O'Brien), against the man's clearly stated wishes. After death, O'Byrne was 'buried' at sea, only for his skeleton to turn up in Hunter's collection a couple of years later. Indeed, O'Byrne's foot bones are visible in the background of one of Hunter's most celebrated portraits and his articulated skeleton remains on display in the Hunterian Museum at the Royal College of Surgeons.

> **Question 1**: Should O'Byrne's wishes finally be heeded and his remains buried, or should his bones be retained as a focus of display and study?

One of the more startling instances of tissue retention concerns Henrietta Lacks (1920–51). Lacks attended the public wards of the Johns Hopkins Medical School Hospital, and presented with vaginal bleeding following her fifth pregnancy. She was treated for cervical cancer and her tumour cells were successfully cultured. This was done without Lacks' knowledge or consent, albeit at a time before the modern concept of informed consent was developed. Although Lacks died quickly, her cell line did not: it is seemingly immortal. Scientists at Johns Hopkins distributed samples of the cells, dubbed 'HeLa', to colleagues throughout the USA. At the present, there are countless trillions of HeLa cells on earth, and the subculture has been used to develop the polio vaccine. The cells have made millions of dollars for biomedical companies. No money has yet been submitted to Lacks' widower or children.

> **Question 2**: Do you think any restitution is owed to the Lacks family or should the individual's story be subordinate to the achievements of successful tissue culture and its therapeutic applications? Does your reaction to the story change when you learn that Lacks was African-American?

A failure to observe the progressively higher standards demanded from the medical profession by the public at large can create problems when long-established practice becomes outmoded and unacceptable. In 1999, for example, a number of English hospitals fell under scrutiny for their routine collection of organs from deceased infants and children. The resulting scandal became particularly associated with the Alder Hey Children's Hospital in Liverpool.

> **Question 3**: Using the Internet, research the events and 'exposés' linked to forensic pathology and the scandal of 1999. Include at least three types of website in your research, including the archive of at least one British newspaper. In your opinion, who or what was most responsible for the public outcry: individual medical practitioners, hospital administrators, the tabloid press, procedural inertia in the NHS or some other factor?

The emergence of ethics in medical research is very recent. It is not too much to claim that a medical career spanning the 1950s to the 1990s would have witnessed a revolution in the way organic human material is gathered.

Why is this relevant?
- Medical research is partly a matter of balancing the rights of the individual patient, the imperatives of inquiry and the mores of society.
- Medical authority was eroded globally over the second half of the twentieth century, partly as a result of the behaviour of medical practitioners and partly due to an increasingly litigious social context.
- Ethics committees and research scrutiny are vital components in the ongoing development of the doctor–patient relationship; *but* rigorous enforcement can reduce drastically the potential progenitors of research (i.e. by ensuring that applications come from large bodies and not from individual practitioners).
- Public opinion can force legal change; among other things, the Human Tissue Act 2004 can trace its origins to the Alder Hey scandal.

Further reading
Skloot R. *The Immortal Life of Henrietta Lacks.* Basingstoke: Macmillan; 2010.

6

Madness and fear

NHS is 'failing' mental health patients

Three-quarters of people suffering from mental illness do not have access to treatments which would improve their lives and save billions of pounds every year, experts warn today.

A damning report, from the London School of Economics and Political Science, says the NHS is failing millions of adults and hundreds of thousands of children with common mental health problems such as anxiety and depression.

N Lakhani, *The Independent*, 18 June 2012

In spite of current criticisms regarding the shortfall in services for the mentally ill, people with mental illness are significantly better treated and accepted now than they have been at any time in the past. Whatever the epoch or culture, society's attitude towards the mentally ill is mostly influenced by prevailing aetiological beliefs. Whereas most people in the contemporary Western world would not regard mental illness as self-inflicted, this has not been always the case. Just like other forms of disability, the early Christian understanding of mental illness was that it represented a punishment for sin (*see* Chapter 2 in this section, 'Two steps forward, one step back: disability') or that the afflicted individual was involuntarily possessed by the devil. An alternative view held by informed medical opinion during the Renaissance was based on humoral theory, which has its roots in Hippocratic medicine of the fourth and fifth centuries BC (*see* Section 6, Chapter 1, 'Early Greek and Roman contributions'). This provided an explanatory scheme for all illness, physical and mental, as well as temperament through an excessive amount of one of the four humours. Thus, too much black bile could result in melancholia whereas too much blood gave rise to mania. Traditional treatments included bloodletting and adherence to specific diets.

During the early Enlightenment a physician and anatomist, Thomas Willis (1621–75), tried to localise mental function to particular parts of the brain. He wrote about this in his book *Cerebri anatome* [The anatomy of the brain] of 1664, in which he termed the study of brain and nerves 'neurologie'. He concluded that 'spirits' travel to and from the heart and brain and, once in the brain, move to the corpus callosum and then the cortex. His book was popular and continued to be read into the nineteenth century. It also marked an important change in conceptualisation of mental illness by firmly framing it as a bodily disorder and therefore possibly responsive to physical cure. The Enlightenment was an intellectually productive time when curious men could be experts in 'natural philosophy' – what we would now regard as science, medicine, art and philosophy. Learned societies established throughout Europe, which provided opportunities for exchange of ideas, presentation of research and collaborative projects. One of the first of these in Britain was that of the Royal Society for Improving Natural Knowledge, which received a Royal Charter in 1662. Non-institutionalised or less formal societies subsequently proliferated. One well known example is that of the Lunar Society in Birmingham, which was established in the 1760s and provided an intellectual space for medicine, contemporary science and technology to meet. The broth of knowledge to be found in such organisations frequently bubbled up to produce exciting new insights.

The story of how behavioural psychology first began illustrates the benefits of cross-disciplinary intercourse. David Hartley (1705–57), who introduced this psychology, was inspired by the ideas of the highly influential philosopher John Locke (1632–1704), expressed in *An Essay Concerning Human Understanding* (1690). Locke, in contrast to René Descartes (1496–1650), did not think that people were born with a ready-made set of logical beliefs. Instead, he proposed that our ideas are shaped by our life experiences and that we have the ability to make associations between our ideas, thereby forming new ideas. Hartley extrapolated this notion to a theory that behaviour could be manipulated by its emotional consequences for the individual. From these thinkers arose the rationale for a new therapeutic intervention – 'moral therapy' for the insane. This approach fundamentally rested on the Lockean recognition that the insane had not 'lost the Faculty of Reasoning' (*Essay on Human Understanding*) but had, by putting the wrong ideas together, come to erroneous conclusions. Further, they were not like animals, who Descartes had described as devoid of soul and reasoning; therefore, the insane should not be treated in a barbaric way. Hartley and another proto-psychologist, John Gay (1685–1732), believed that rewards and punishments could be used to shape behaviour, thereby rehabilitating the individual. This new 'psychology' proved to be influential in a number of social public settings such as schools, factories and prisons (*see* Section 4, Chapter 7, 'Child welfare'). Moral management of the insane was adopted by some of the more enlightened and humane 'private' madhouse keepers such as Thomas Bakewell (1761–1835), who in 1808 established a madhouse called Spring Vale, and a Quaker family in York called Tuke. William Tuke (1732–1822) developed the York Retreat (from 1796) in response to the appalling conditions of the asylum at York in which a Quaker woman had died. Private madhouses were diverse in comfort, size and the skills of the proprietors. In response to their variability, the Madhouses Act 1774 was passed, introducing licensing, inspection by magistrates and supervision by a physician. Significantly, there was no direction to cure in this act. Further, the legislation did not apply to the public asylums or privately boarded 'single luna-tics', nor did it impose penalties for infringements.

Until about 1800, most of the poor insane were sent to workhouses to work, as a result of the Poor Relief Act 1601. The Vagrancy Act of 1744 differentiated 'vagrants' – that is, people who were found outside their parish without permis-sion – in such a way that now those who were considered 'lunatics' could be sent to special accommodation for possible 'cure' instead of houses of detention; this is the first reference made to an aspiration to cure, although no suggestion is made about how this might be achieved. This act reveals the process by which the poor insane were admitted and discharged: only local magistrates could determine the presence of insanity, not doctors, and once an insane person was locked up in 'some secure place', they remained there until they were deemed 'recovered' by the magistrate or jailer.

The early nineteenth century saw active reformist legislative change. In 1808, the County Asylums Act established the principle that the local population should pay taxes to establish asylums for the care of the poor lunatic. By 1845, this became mandatory. The intention had been to establish institutions run on moral therapy lines, which were well staffed, regulated and inspected. Indeed, some excellent models existed, such as The (1st Middlesex) County Asylum at Hanwell. Hanwell, built in 1831 and set on 74 acres, was the first purpose-built asylum for the poor insane. It was self-sufficient, cultivating its own produce and having its own bakery, laundry, gasworks, fire brigade, dock and even a brewery. Its third medical superintendent was the enlightened John Conolly (1794–1866), an active campaigner for moral therapy and non-restraint. However, by the second half of the century, the picture had changed. Asylums had become overcrowded repositories for anyone considered socially deviant. By 1900, there were 77 asylums housing at least 80 000 people. They had once again become places for confinement not cure.

Mentally ill patients were often treated appallingly, as the Lancet Commission described in its report *The Care and Cure of the Insane* in 1877: 'Everywhere attendants, we are convinced, maltreat, abuse and terrify patients when the backs of the medical officers are turned. Humanity is only secured by watching officials.' Further, according to the report, conditions were very poor: clothing was 'torn and dirty', lavatories 'very defective' and the corridors 'meagre'.

The only medicines available were chloral hydrate and opium. With so little prospect of cure, therapeutic nihilism set in, supported by the popular non-Darwinian theory of hereditary degeneration, which asserted that insanity becomes increasingly extreme as it is passed down the generations. Such beliefs resulted in stigma and fuelled a prejudice that the mentally ill had no value in society. By the second half of the nineteenth century, the pendulum of public opinion had swung back to a more intolerant and fearful position. While the newspapers then, as now, tended to be sensationalist, they also reflected public attitudes:

'The present laws . . . protect the liberty of the lunatic at the expense of the lives, limbs and comfort . . . of the sane' (A Lunatic's Victim, Letter, *The Times*, 23 May 1877). There were also worries that sane individuals might be mistakenly detained, an issue that had been identified by the 1877 Commission, and this was reflected in the popular literature: '[A]ny attempt to rescue her by legal means would, even if successful, involve a delay which might be fatal to her . . . intellect, which is already shaken by the horror of the situation to which she has been confined' (W Collins, *The Woman in White*, 1869). These concerns were addressed by the Lunacy Act of 1890, which concentrated on protecting the public from illegal detention and did little to support asylums in becoming places of cure rather than containment.

Following the emergence of a movement for deinstitutionalisation and community care in the 1950s and 1960s, all the large asylums for the mentally ill were gradually closed. Beds were dramatically reduced and specially designed hospital units were built for those who required admission. The distinction between mental hospitals and general hospitals was removed by the Mental Health Act 1959, so psychiatric units could be located in general hospitals. The discovery of antipsychotics and antidepressants in the 1950s brought a new therapeutic optimism to the management of people with severe mental illness and reduced the need for long admissions (*see* Section 7, Chapter 3, 'The rise of pharmacology: a story of prepared minds, money and serendipity'). Community care provided the opportunity for people to live more autonomously and normally. Although this has been the case for many, today others find themselves socially isolated, ghettoised and without any meaningful activity to do. While community mental health and social workers try to mitigate this, they often fight a losing battle against economic cuts.

Despite the progress made in understanding and treating mental illness, sufferers continued to be stigmatised, even ill-treated. During the Second World War, over 70 000 were gassed by Nazis as a result of the eugenics movement. The list of victims was drawn up by physicians, including psychiatrists. These days, the public's preoccupying fear concerning the mentally ill is that of violence, as the following quotation illustrates:

> Movies and other forms of popular entertainment often present misinformation about and negative portrayals of schizophrenia, which can lead to confused public opinion, new research suggests. In a review of more than 40 contemporary movies that depict characters with schizophrenia, researchers found that most of the characters showed violent behavior, almost one third showed homicidal behaviour, and one fourth committed suicide.
>
> D Brauser, Schizophrenia in the movies, *Medscape Today* [website],
> 4 September 2012

Why is this relevant?

- Although 'madness' is a part of the human condition, the sane have always tried to put social and conceptual distance between themselves and the insane.
- In spite of deinstitutionalisation and the advent of many effective treatments, the public of the twenty-first century, like those of previous centuries, remains distrustful and fearful of the mentally ill.
- Although many thought that closing down asylums and 'normalising' the mentally ill were laudable aims, the reality is that many now live on their own in cheap housing, isolated and under-employed. Is this so humane?

Further reading

Porter R. *Enlightenment: Britain and the creation of the modern world.* London: Penguin; 2000.

Porter R. *Madness: a brief history.* Oxford: Oxford University Press; 2002.

Porter R. *Mind Forg'd Manacles: a history of madness in England from the Restoration to the Regency.* London: Penguin; 1987.

Uglow J. *The Lunar Men: the friends who made the future.* London: Faber and Faber; 2003.

Zimmer C. *Soul Made Flesh: the discovery of the brain – and how it changed the world.* London: Heinemann; 2004.

7

Mind and brain

Tell me where is fancie bred,
Or in the heart, or in the head?

Shakespeare, *The Merchant of Venice*,
Act 3, Scene 2, lines 63–4

DEBATE ABOUT THE LOCATION OF THE MIND HAS EXTENDED FROM AT least the time of Ancient Greece to the Renaissance, and some would contend that it is still a matter of controversy today. Aristotle (384–322 BC) was quite convinced that the heart was the site of thought and emotions, and that the brain's function was to cool the heart to which it was connected. Hippocrates (c. 460–c. 370 BC) was of the opinion that the brain was the site of intelligence. Debate continued into Renaissance Europe and spread to the Arab world. The influential physician Avicenna (980–1037 AD) combined the above views by proposing that sensations, cognition and movement were the function of the brain but that the brain was controlled by the heart. This 'hedging of bets' is amusingly illustrated in *One Thousand and One Nights* [Kitāb alf laylah wa-laylah] by Scheherazade's response on her four hundred and thirty-ninth night of telling stories to amuse the king to save her life, to a question on the location of the seat of understanding: 'Allah casteth it in the heart whence its illustrious beams ascend to the brain and there become fixed.'

Galen (129–c. 200 AD), who had dissected animals but not humans, believed that the brain was the source of thought and that 'animal spirits' were housed in the brain's ventricles. Because he was so influential, his many misunderstandings of human anatomy were not contested until the sixteenth century, when Andreas Vesalius (1514–64), a Flemish physician and anatomist, wrote *De humani corporis fabrica libri septem* [On the fabric of the human body in seven books] in 1543. He had been given the right to dissect executed criminals while a professor in Padua. Leonardo Da Vinci also produced some very accurate descriptions of the brain, particularly in the late sixteenth century, when he had access to cadavers for dissection. In spite of these excellent physical descriptions, there was still little understanding of the function of the brain until Thomas Willis (1621–75) published *Cerebri anatome* [The anatomy of the brain] in 1664, which was closely followed by Nicolas Steno's (1638–86) *Lecture on the Anatomy of the Brain* in

1669 [Discours de M. Steno sur L'anatomie du cerveau]. Both were highly critical of Galen.

Another debate that caused considerable controversy was that of the location of the soul. René Descartes (1596–1650), who had studied the anatomy of the brain, proposed a theory of 'mind–body dualism'; that is, a separation between a material body (brain) and immaterial mind (soul). Rather unconvincingly, he sited the soul in the pineal gland because, he argued, there had to be a mechanism by which a material brain could communicate with an immaterial soul/mind. Physicians who specialised in mental illness embraced this new materialism, since it allowed them to explain mental illness as a disorder of a material brain. They were not obliged to discuss the role or place of the soul/mind, so could avoid ecclesiastical dispute.

> **Discussion point**: Discuss contemporary views regarding the location and nature of the mind. Do we have it pinned down to our satisfaction?

Sigmund Freud (1856–1939), who was originally trained as a neurologist, thought that the mind was reducible to the brain. However, his theories about the unconscious mind made no reference to neurological substrates. Psychoanalysis proved very popular and dominated psychiatry, especially in North America, for at least the first half of the twentieth century. Freud's theories brought a new explanatory model of how the mind works, and his theories spawned a number of different psychotherapies over the ensuing decades. So influential were the theories of Freud and his protégés that many of their concepts concerning how we mentally function are now well integrated into popular culture.

> **Question**: Can you think of some examples?

A neuroscientific model for understanding the brain took much longer to gain popular and professional appeal. Its beginnings can be traced back to the nineteenth century. Carl Wernicke (1848–1905) worked on localisation of brain function, particularly with regard to language. The German neuropathologist and psychiatrist Alois Alzheimer (1864–1915) described the clinical presentation of dementia and in 1906 succeeded in linking it with specific pathological findings in the brain. Thirty years later, neuroscientific understanding, albeit often flawed, began to lead to some physical treatments for specific disorders.

First, there was Manfred Sakel (1900–57) in Vienna, who introduced insulin-induced coma in 1933 to treat schizophrenia, apparently with some success. Another new treatment for schizophrenia was introduced by a doctor from Budapest, Ladislas J Meduna (1896–1964) – cardiazol-induced seizures. This intervention was based on the erroneous hypothesis that schizophrenia and epilepsy were antagonistic diseases. William Sargant (1907–88), a psychiatrist who worked at the Maudsley Hospital in London, noticed that the seizures seemed to work best for depressive symptoms and tried it out successfully on patients with depressive disorder. Around the same time, Ugo Cerletti (1877–1963) from Genoa, Italy, began using electric shock treatment to treat severe depression. In the USA, leucotomy, which was introduced by Egas Moniz (1874–1955), became popular through the efforts of an American neurologist, Walter Freeman II (1895–1972), who refined this operation. The technique involved severing the connections between the frontal lobes and the rest of the brain. By 1951, over 18 000 patients in the USA had undergone leucotomy, by which time some of its drawbacks and failures were becoming apparent.

Such treatments seem crude to contemporary eyes and indeed came in for significant criticism from the anti-psychiatry movement in later years. But at that time, there were no other effective treatments available (antipsychotics and antidepressants had not yet been developed) and the psychiatric wards were full of patients with little hope of improvement. As Sargant relates in his book *The Unquiet Mind* (1967), '[i]t distressed us when people came begging us to take relatives of theirs into our hospital for the new treatments [that] were forbidden by the hospitals to which their dear ones had been admitted'. He continues to describe his experiences of visiting a ward of another hospital with his 'shock-box', which contained

> more than forty of those unfortunates [suffering with agitated depression], one of whom screamed at me to get out. She said that I had sent her there from the Maudsley two years previously and she had been given no treatment ever since ... We gave nearly the whole ward of agitated depressives the new electric shock treatment. More than thirty made a quick recovery and were soon able to leave hospital. Yet I admit that ... our sending an electric current through the patient's head was always an anxious event for us.

In 1944, Sargant and Eliot Slater published *An Introduction to Physical Methods of Treatments in Psychiatry*, several editions of which would go on to be published in the following decades. Sargant recalls that 10 years previously, while he was working at The (1st Middlesex) County Asylum at Hanwell, there were few physical treatments available: '[E]xcept for malaria fever treatment of brain syphilis and such old crude sedatives as bromides, medinal and paraldehyde, few other physical treatments for mental illness were known'. This was all soon to change with the discovery of chlorpromazine in 1952, the mood stabiliser lithium in 1949 and the antidepressant imipramine, which was launched in 1958; it took a few more years to appreciate the mode of action of these drugs.

This chemical revolution contributed to two developments. One was the legitimisation of the neuroscientific model and consequently the gradual demise of psychoanalysis. The other was the reduction of institutional care. There continues to be debate over how important the latter was to the creation of the new policy to close the asylums and transfer care to the community; the emerging anti-psychiatry movement and the costs of maintaining huge asylums for the NHS were also factors in this.

The emergence of magnetic resonance imaging and positron emission tomography has further progressed our understanding of human behaviour and emotions. Many neuroscientists regard the human mind or consciousness as a purely biological process. This has caused controversy, especially among those interested in moral, religious and philosophical considerations of human consciousness.

In Benjamin Kunkel's fictional book *Indecision* (2005), the protagonist suffers with permanent indecision for which he is offered a cure called 'abulinex'. He ponders the implications of this miracle cure: 'abulinex would force me to decide that my entire personality boiled down to neurochemistry, and I only flattered myself I possessed a freewill'.

Why is this relevant?

- The discourse that took place from the seventeenth century on the location of the soul/mind has been revitalised, although we are more likely to substitute the word 'mind' or 'consciousness' for 'soul'. The debate on this subject is often vitriolic, just as it was centuries ago. The Judeo-Christian religions differentiated the human race from animals on the basis of the belief that only humans possessed a soul. Indeed, one of the rationalisations for not treating the mentally ill with respect and dignity in the past was that they had descended to the state of beasts. Many contemporary scientists would rest the distinction between humans and animals on the presence in humans of a higher consciousness. Something about our specialness seems to be very much at stake here. This seems to be not only about asserting our uniqueness among all living organisms but also about a strong dislike of the notion that our 'higher' mental events and emotional states could be reduced to chemical events in our brain.

- Massive scale institutionalisation of the mentally ill seems to have come and gone. However, just like 'care in the community', asylum care for the mentally ill was initially perceived as reformist and laudable. Both approaches were initially greeted with enthusiasm that time has diminished.

- New treatments do not always fulfil their promise. Just as leucotomy and the first-generation antipsychotics were hailed as breakthroughs, so were serotonin reuptake inhibitors (antidepressants) and atypical antipsychotics. None of these is completely effective or devoid of problems.

- In the past, new treatments were used experimentally on the most vulnerable in ways that might now be regarded as cavalier. This is far less likely to occur now, given the requirements of research ethics committees. However, doctors like Sargant were motivated by compassion and a desire to cure, and their forthright approach may not only have benefited individuals but also led to a more rapid acceptance of more effective treatments.

Further reading

Braslow J. *Mental Ills and Bodily Cures: psychiatric treatments in the first half of the twentieth century.* Berkley and Los Angeles, CA, and London: University of California Press; 1997.

Gay P. *Freud: a life for our time*. London: J M Dent; 1987.

Porter R. *Madness: a brief history*. Oxford: Oxford University Press; 2002.

Sargant W. *The Unquiet Mind*. London: Heinemann; 1967.

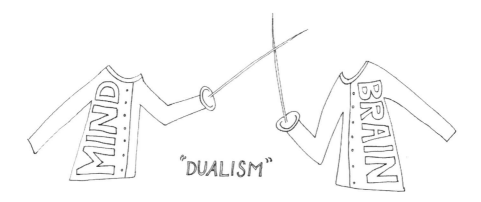

Section 6

Practising medicine: diagnostic methods

1

Early Greek and Roman contributions

THE PROCESS OF DIAGNOSIS RELIES ON HOLDING A MODEL OF ILLNESS that informs the health practitioner of possible causes. The study of the history of medicine shows us how frameworks of understanding disease have changed over millennia to bring us to our current position. During that journey, certain epochs and places stand out as times of significant medical progress. Great men and women are often perceived as the catalysts of progress, yet such people rarely appear spontaneously. They are products of their time; the acceptance of their ideas often is dependent on simultaneous progress in other disciplines. Hippocrates (c. 460–c. 370 BC) is often called the father of medicine for very good reasons, but his spirit of inquiry came at a time of significant progress in many disciplines such as Greek theatre, philosophy, astronomy, historiography and mathematics; new ideas in one discipline were noted by other disciplines, tried and elaborated or discarded. That time is now known as the period of Hellenic civilisation.

To appreciate fully the Hippocratic school's contribution to medical science, we have to set aside our current medical understanding and try to imagine how our predecessors made sense of symptoms. In other words, how they identified, evaluated, classified and treated them, given their limited knowledge of the anatomy and physiology of the human body. An analogy would be that of seeing an aeroplane fly for the first time without any knowledge of physics. How would you explain this phenomenon? It is easy for us to denigrate past medical theories (*see* Section 7, Chapter 2, 'Medical misdirection'), but how could these sensibly evolve without a developing body of knowledge in subjects such as anatomy, physiology and microbiology? There was indeed quite a significant corpus of medical knowledge present in civilisations before the Hellenic, largely reliant on handed-down experience, which entered folk or domestic medical practices. It was experience that led the Hebrews to introduce dietary instructions and social and personal hygiene measures, the Hindus to develop certain surgical operations such as rhinoplasty and the Chinese to become experts on herbal medicines. But theories on why treatments worked were limited.

As a broad generalisation, until 600 BC, medical doctrines were based on religious or magical beliefs. Then a new discipline of philosophy emerged that stimulated critical questioning and change by introducing rational reasoning to explain natural phenomena, including disease. This was the Pythagorean school of philosophy. Pythagoras (c. 580–c. 498 BC) is credited with developments in mathematics and music. One of his pupils who also practised medicine, Empedocles (490–430 BC), held that everything in the universe, including humankind, was composed of four 'roots'; these were later renamed by Plato as 'elements'. Empedocles defined their characteristics after the Greek gods thereby revealing that prevailing religious beliefs were still influential. Thus, he describes fire as 'shining Zeus', air as 'life-bringing Hera', earth as Aidoneus or Hades, and water as Nestis, who 'with tears moistens mortal spring' (On Nature and Purifications). These four elements were qualitatively different but in equilibrium and able to unite and separate according to a power battle between the two forces of love and strife. We not only shared the same constituent elements as nature but were subject to the same laws. This doctrine, which is characterised by the privileging of the number four, provided the assumptions on which the humoral theory of health and illness is based. Hippocratic medicine was influenced by these philosophical ideas and embraced humoral theory.

Over ensuing centuries, the humoral theory was elaborated but remained relatively unchanged. It became the authoritative model of health and disease until the nineteenth century thanks to the dogmatic teachings of the physician Galen (129–c. 200 AD), and accounts for the popularity of interventions such as bloodletting. The theory regards the body as being composed of four humours, black bile, yellow bile, phlegm and blood, which echo the four universal elements and the qualities of the four seasons. When in equilibrium and harmony, the state of 'eucrasia' (health) is established; disequilibrium and 'dyscrasia' (disharmony) lead to disease. Many environmental factors could cause disequilibrium, including the weather, the season or diet. Treatment rested on restoring equilibrium such as by countering an excess of humour with its opposite. For example, the hot dry state of a fever caused by an excess of yellow bile might be treated with phlegm using cold baths. Alternatively, an excess of a particular humour could be managed by means such as vomiting, voiding or bloodletting, depending on the offending humour. Diagnosis was a tricky business because factors such as the predominant humour of the individual when in good health (indicated by their temperament) had to be taken into account as well as the effects of the environment. Thus, a meticulous medical history, complemented by good clinical observation, was essential.

Question: Are there any examples in current biomedical knowledge of the number four being significant?

THE FOUR HUMOURS

Quality	Season	Humour	Organ	Element	Temperament
Cold and dry	Autumn	Black bile	Liver	Earth	Melancholic
Hot and moist	Spring	Blood	Heart	Air	Sanguine
Cold and moist	Winter	Phlegm	Brain	Water	Phlegmatic
Hot and dry	Summer	Yellow bile	Spleen	Fire	Choleric

Hippocrates was thought to be a descendant of Aesculapius (c. 1250 BC) who was a great healer and deified after his death. People worshipped Aesculapius in temples called *asclepieia*, where they attended for the healing ritual 'temple sleep', which was facilitated by snakes – this is why the British Medical Association's logo depicts him with staff entwined by a snake. Remains of these temples can be seen today at places such as Epidaurus, Cos and Athens. The Hippocratic Collection consists of a number of works, which were probably written over a period of 200 years and by several authors who followed the Hippocratic method. They include a code of ethics, the Hippocratic Oath, which remains relevant to modern practice. The clinical texts are characterised by thorough clinical observation and logical reasoning. Supernatural or divine causes are discounted in favour of natural causes, which disturb the individual's humoral equilibrium. Emphasis is put on first allowing nature to heal, with the judicious use of diet and baths when necessary. Treatments are tailored to the time of year and take account of the patient's temperament. If the non-invasive 'let nature take its course' method does not work, then a hierarchical approach is advocated, starting with hellebore to induce vomiting and diarrhoea, then the knife (bloodletting), followed by fire (cauterisation) to burn the skin to allow excess humour to drain out.

The study of prognosis was encouraged: 'I hold that it is an excellent thing for the physician to practice forecasting. He will carry out treatment best if he knows beforehand from the present symptoms what will take place later' (*Hippocratic Collection*). One of the most famous books in the Collection is *Aphorisms*, which is full of interesting assertions informed by careful observation of the epidemiology as well as effects of disease. Here are some examples:

- Life is short, and the Art long; opportunity fleeting; experiment dangerous, and judgment difficult.
- All diseases occur at all seasons, but some are more apt to occur and to be aggravated at certain seasons.
- Do not disturb a patient either during or just after a crisis, and try no experiments, neither with purges nor with other irritants, but leave him alone.
- In every disease it is a good sign when the patient's intellect is sound and he enjoys his food; the opposite is a bad sign.
- Old men generally have less illness than young men, but such complaints as become chronic in old men generally last until death.
- Both sleep and sleeplessness when beyond due measure, constitute disease.

- Those diseases that medicines do not cure are cured by the knife. Those that the knife does not cure are cured by fire. Those that fire does not cure must be considered incurable.

Significantly, the Hippocratic method focused full attention on the patient, taking into account his or her symptoms as well as his or her temperament and the environmental circumstances. Today, we would call this 'holistic' medicine.

The Hippocratic was not the only approach to healing. Other schools also flourished, such as that of Knidos, although there, every symptom was classified as a disease. Asclepiades of Bithynia (c. 124 or 129–40 BC), who brought Greek medicine to the Romans in the second century BC, completely rejected elemental and humoral theory as well as the notion of a benevolent nature. Instead, he held that the body was composed of *corpuscula* (molecules) made of *anarmoi ongoi* (atoms) and that irregular distribution of the patient's molecules led to disease. He advocated gentle treatment methods using massage, hydrotherapy, exercise and herbal medicines. His approach was sympathetic and caring, particularly towards the mentally ill, whom he thought would benefit from occupation, music therapy and a good diet.

Asclepiades had worked at the medical school of Alexandria, which was founded in 332 BC. Two of its previous physicians, Erasistratus (304–250 BC) and Herophilus (c. 330–280 BC), deserve mention for the advances they made in anatomical knowledge due to ready access to human corpses for dissection. Although their writings have been lost, we have some idea of their discoveries from subsequent physicians such as Galen. Herophilus performed extensive dissections of the brain and was certain that this was the seat of intelligence. Erasistratus distinguished sensory from motor nerves and the cerebrum from the cerebellum.

Although Galen recognised the importance of anatomy, his dissections were of animals, since human dissection had become illegal by his time. For the next 1500 years, it proved difficult to dissect because of the Christian church's opposition to this practice; this naturally held back knowledge about how the body functioned. However, further progress was primarily delayed by the collapse of the Roman Empire in the fifth century AD. Fortunately, many of the medical books written by Galen had been transcribed by physicians who resided at the new capital of the Roman Empire, Byzantium (Constantinople), and by church scribes. Following the conquest of much of the Roman Empire by followers of Mohammed, these texts were translated into Arabic and then informed Islamic medicine. They later returned to the West through translations from Arabic. Thus, early medical schools, such as that at Salerno in Southern Italy, became well acquainted with Galenic doctrine.

Why is this relevant?

- When a doctor or other clinician practises, they should be aware that their decision-making framework is informed by their model of illness, which has risen from historical and philosophical influences.
- A spirit of inquiry and a cross-disciplinary approach are as important today as they were in the past to foster new ideas.
- Progress is facilitated by people who are prepared to think unconventionally and creatively and to engage with new ideas and different disciplines.
- How vulnerable is our corpus of medical knowledge today to natural or manufactured disasters?

Further reading

Guthrie D. *A History of Medicine.* London: Thomas Nelson; 1945.

van Der Eijk P. Medicine and health in the Graeco-Roman world. In: Jackson M, editor. *The Oxford Handbook of The History of Medicine.* Oxford and New York, NY: Oxford University Press; 2011. pp. 21–39.

2

'[T]he most liquid evacuations imaginable': excreta as a diagnostic tool

THE QUOTE IN THE CHAPTER TITLE COMES FROM A LETTER WRITTEN by Susanna Darwin, the mother of Charles Darwin, in a letter to her brother Josiah Wedgwood; and, yes, she is describing her bowel movements. This level of honesty in a letter to a sibling is startling to modern sensibilities; we would be unlikely to use this tone or go into this much detail with anyone other than our partner, and perhaps even not then. If we did, we might invite an accusation of 'sharing too much'. But the state of one's bowels was a constant preoccupation for people prior to the more repressed Victorian era, and little wonder – faeces do not have to be bloody to be of interest.

The scrutinising of both urine and faeces was integral to diagnostic technique prior to 1800. Doctors of all descriptions would ask for samples of both excretions and would make recommendations about diagnosis and treatment based on visual examination, smell and, in the case of urine, taste. The qualities of a person's faeces were thought to be intimately bound (no pun intended) to their state of mind. This explains why, in Nicholas Hytner's film *The Madness of King George* (1994), the King's physicians take particular pains to analyse his poo, giving rise to both speculation and scepticism. As one character puts it to another, 'one can produce a copious, regular and exquisitely turned evacuation every day of the week and still be a stranger to reason.' Nonetheless, patients admitted to lunatic asylums in nineteenth-century England routinely had their bowel movements monitored and noted in superintendents' casebooks.

The experience of evacuation was also of intense interest to patients. In an era when the poor had a very limited dietary range and the rich a very extensive one that was nonetheless short in fibre, constipation could be more than just a pain in the bum. Haemorrhoids were just the start. Surgeons routinely undertook the treatment of anal fistulae, caused by the strain on the tissues around the rectum that had become so great that hard faeces had channelled a new path to the outside of the body. This was, in a period prior to effective painkillers, an excruciating complaint and could only be treated by the new channel being sewn up and the faeces after the operation being rendered as liquid as possible for a period of healing.

Question 1: How are anal fistulae managed today?

The consistency of stools over a period of time remains of concern, if only in the very private arena. Self-appointed advisors such as health-shop personnel speak in anodyne terms of obtaining sufficient dietary fibre, and advertisements for nutritional supplements allude to 'bloating' and friendly bacteria in the gut. However, there is a serious public health issue concerning illnesses in which the opposite affliction – watery diarrhoea – is a symptom.

Question 2: Why is this? What illnesses are characterised by this symptom?

In twenty-first-century Britain, sensibilities are being challenged more robustly by a public campaign urging people to see their general practitioner (GP) if they experience a significant or sustained change in their stools or bowel habit (in other words, the frequency with which they defecate and any notable change in the consistency of their excreta). It uses idiomatic language rather than clinical terms to engage more successfully with the lay public.

Why is this relevant?

- Patients, particularly new mothers, the costive and older people, may regard purgatives as a vital component of their daily comfort. This is not a trivial matter but the difference between constant, low-level pain and relief.

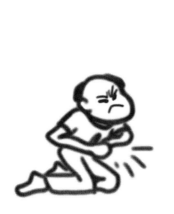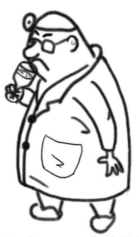

—— Your urine looks clear, its bouquet is full-bodied and it tastes well, so there can't be anything wrong with you!

- The reticent may be significantly averse to confessing to any digestive or anal discomfort, so may have to be prompted sensitively. At its most drastic, such inhibition may delay investigation of bowel polyps or abrasions, but it can also have more chronic implications if the presenting issue is not sensitively teased out.
- Excreta remain a diagnostic aid in the cases of the very young, older people, people experiencing significant challenges to communication and in poor societies in which investigative tests are not available.

3

The rise of modern medicine: the evolution of modern physical diagnosis

MOST ORDINARY PHYSICIANS OF THE RENAISSANCE DISDAINED physically examining their patients. What was the necessity when you knew that disease was a matter of humoral imbalance? A careful account would tell you the temperament of your patient: sanguineous, melancholic, phlegmatic or choleric, dependent on which of the four humours predominated (respectively blood, black bile, phlegm or yellow bile). These interacted with the four elements: air, fire, earth and water, and the four qualities of heat, cold, moisture and dryness. Each person's disease resulted from unique imbalances and interactions of these humours, elements and qualities. So, diagnosis was an intellectual activity reliant on a careful history helped by certain observations, such as your patient's skin pallor and the constitution of her or his urine and excreta. When this is your model of disease, there is no need to know anything else about the inside of your patient's body.

The modern approach to medicine was ushered in slowly by a paradigm shift in the conceptualisation of disease. This shift was possible due to certain technical advances and a number of free-thinking men, although many other factors set the stage for progress.

- Thanks to a relaxation of restriction on human dissection, Andreas Vesalius (1514–64) provided accurate anatomical knowledge on which physical diagnosis could be based in his *De humani corporis fabrica libri septem* (1543).
- Thomas Sydenham's (1624–89) obsessional clinical observations allowed him to provide accurate descriptions of each disease. He then attempted to define, classify and name them all and published a book, *Methodus curandi febres* [The method of curing fevers] on the new method – 'nosology' – in 1666. In contrast, François Boissier de Sauvages de Lacroix (1706–67) chose symptoms as the basis for disease classification, which led to him describing 2400 'diseases', including 19 types of dysphagia and 18 types of angina. He failed to see the difference between a symptom and a syndrome.
- William Harvey (1578–1657) provided the basis of modern physiology with

his soundly argued and experimentally supported exposition of how the heart works (*see* the next chapter in this section, 'The beat, beat, beat of the drum: the discovery of circulation and the tools to measure it').

- Giovanni Battista Morgagni (1682–1771) established the idea that whole organs could be diseased. Not only did he describe pathological changes in minute detail with the aid of a microscope, but he also linked these findings to the patient's history, symptoms and treatment. His publication *De Sedibus et Causis Morborum per Anatomen Indagatis* [The seats and causes of diseases as investigated by anatomy] (1761) represented a lifetime of research.

- Philippe Pinel (1745–1826) grouped diseases by tissue rather than anatomical location, such as all diseases of the mucous membranes in his *Nosologie Philosophique ou Méthode de l'Analyse Appliquée à la Médecine* [Nosology and philosophical analysis method applied to medicine] (1798). This was a completely new method of categorisation. Marie François Xavier Bichat (1771–1802) expanded on this concept by describing the symptoms that arose from the diseased tissue and the dysfunction of the organ involved.

- Bedside teaching was introduced by Hermann Boerhaave (1668–1738) at Leyden from 1700. He had access to 12 beds and used these to teach students from all over Europe. He insisted that students attend post-mortems and made them link the clinical findings prior to death with those on post-mortem.

Boerhaave's clinical observations were limited to observation and examination of the pulse and bodily products. At this time, there were no techniques or instruments to ascertain the state of a diseased organ in a living patient. Then Leopold Auenbrugger (1722–1809), an innkeeper's son with an ear for music, 'opened up the world of the ear as a clinical instrument'. He became a physician and while working in Vienna discovered that he could use percussion to differentiate between a healthy and diseased organ. His technique involved striking the chest covered by a tight shirt with the tips of two extended fingers held close together during normal breathing and then inspiration and expiration. He differentiated four notes – normal, tympanic, dull, and flat – and went on to describe the sounds he elicited for different lung diseases as well as those in dropsy and aneurysm: 'If a sonorous region of the chest appears, on percussion, entirely destitute of the natural sounds – that is, if it yields only a sound like that of a fleshy limb when struck – disease exists in that region.' His book, 'A new discovery that enables the physician from the percussion of the human thorax to detect the diseases hidden in the chest' [Latin], published in 1761, received little interest. Matters may have been different had Morgagni's book on pathological anatomy, which was published in the same year, had been well known. However, Jean-Nicolas Corvisart (1755–1821), France's most well-respected physician at the time, brought percussion into mainstream French clinical practice through translating Auenbrugger's book into French and describing the process in his own textbook in 1806. The method was not used outside France until popularised by René Laennec (1781–1826), who was a former pupil of Corvisart. In 1819, Laennec published a two-volume study called *De l'Auscultation Mediate* [On mediate auscultation] discussing the use of the stethoscope.

Laennec's development of the stethoscope was described by a friend:

> The author told me himself, the great discovery which has immortalised his name was due to chance...One day walking in the court of the Louvre, he saw some children, who, with their ears glued to the two ends of some long pieces of wood which transmitted the sound of the little blows of the pins, struck at the opposite end...He conceived instantly the thought of applying this to the study of diseases of the heart. On the morrow, at his clinic at the Necker Hospital, he took a sheet of paper, rolled it up, tied it with a string, making a central canal which he then placed on a diseased heart. This was the first stethoscope.
>
> Major RH. *A History of Medicine.* Springfield: Charles C Thomas; 1954. pp. 661–2.

Laennec had been using direct auscultation for some years by putting the ear directly to the chest. He disliked this method for its impracticality and indelicacy; women often refused to accept it. In subsequent years, he experimented with different designs of stethoscope, making these instruments himself. His favourite was 45 cm long, 4 cm wide and could be disassembled into two parts for portability.

The rest of the nineteenth century witnessed the development of several instruments used to facilitate physical examination and bedside diagnosis, such as the ophthalmoscope in 1850, the thermometer in 1871 and reflex hammer in 1875 to elicit deep tendon reflexes.

Question: Who developed these instruments and what reception did they have?

In 1895, X-rays were discovered by a German physicist, Wilhelm Röntgen (1845–1923). The possibility of visualising and taking photographs of the denser materials within a human being captured the public's imagination. Fears that people's intimate areas would be visible led one underwear company to advertise his products as X-ray proof! It seems that certain fears are recurrent, as similar concerns have emerged recently in reaction to security scanners at airports, as the following headline attests: 'Inventor creates X-ray proof underpants to protect modesty of passengers in 'naked' airport scanners' (Y Qureshi, *Manchester Evening News* [online], 15 March 2011).

Why is this relevant?

- Most religions value the sanctity of the human body. Therefore, it is not surprising that human dissection was disapproved of and frequently outlawed across different cultures and epochs. This had the effect of impeding the understanding of human anatomy and physiology, thereby delaying medical progress. Medical endeavour can be still constrained by religious doctrine, for example, as it has been in the field of human embryonic stem cell research.

- Medical investigative procedures mushroomed once Galenic teachings were abandoned in favour of a model of illness based on a proper understanding of human anatomy and physiology.
- Each investigative procedure has required the development of new medical skills, from auscultation to interpretation of magnetic resonance images. Arguably, some skills become almost redundant as investigative procedures become more automated.

Further reading

Walker HK. The origins of the history and physical examination. In: Walker HK, Hall WD, Hurst JW, editors. *Clinical Methods: the history, physical and laboratory examination*. 3rd ed. Boston, MA: Butterworths; 1990. Available at: www.ncbi.nlm.nih.gov/books/NBK458/ (accessed 21 April 2013).

4

The beat, beat, beat of the drum: the discovery of circulation and the tools to measure it

IT MAY SEEM STRANGE TO US LIVING IN THE TWENTY-FIRST CENTURY that an erroneous understanding of the function of the heart and blood persisted for 1500 years. The favoured paradigm had rested on Galenic teaching and was not overturned until 1628, when William Harvey (1578–1657) published *Exercitatio Anatomica de Motu Cordis et Sanguinis in Animalibus* [An anatomical exercise on the motion of the heart and blood in living beings] in which he demonstrated that the heart was a pump and drove blood around the body. Galen (129–c. 200 AD) thought that the liver produced blood, which was carried around the body by blood vessels. He was aware that the blood in arteries was brighter than that carried in the veins and considered this to be due to 'pneuma' (air) that had been absorbed from the lung into the pulmonary veins. According to this theory, blood did not circulate but ebbed and flowed. On reaching the end of a vein or artery, blood and air were released to the local tissues according to how much was needed. He also wrongly thought that blood could pass to the left side of the heart through pores in the ventricular septum.

Before Galen, there was very little understanding of the function of blood vessels, let alone the heart; however, the pulse rate had engaged the attention of physicians of antiquity. According to the *Ebers Papyrus* (c. 1550 BC), it seems that Egyptians felt the pulse to evaluate a patient's condition and realised that it was synchronous with the heartbeat. It is unlikely that they measured it, because they had no instruments that could measure small units of time. Some 1200 years later, the Greek physician Herophilus (335–280 BC), who was a leading physician at the famous medical school in Alexandria, was able to measure the pulse using a water clock. His access to cadavers for dissection and criminals for experiments furnished him with unique anatomical insights for the time. He concluded that arteries and veins had different functions and that the pulse could be felt only in arteries. Galen was acquainted with some of his work but criticised his 'scientific' approach – that is, learning based on experimentation and observation. While Galen was developing his reputation, the most famous surgeon in China,

Hua Tuo (140–208 AD), was making a thorough study of the pulse, which he believed could be used to diagnose any internal illness. A long lull in progress ensued but for Gilles de Corbeil's (c. 1200 AD) poem in hexameter on the pulse, *De Pulsibus* [On pulses]; he was a French physician who had graduated from the famous Salerno School of Medicine. In addition, the pulmonary circulation was described by Ibn al-Nafis (1213–88 AD), who speculated that there must be small 'pores' between the ends of the pulmonary vein and artery; these were identified as capillaries about 400 years later by Marcello Malpighi (1628–94) using a new invention, the microscope (*see* the next chapter in this section, 'From toy to tool: the microscope').

William Harvey lived at a time of significant intellectual activity. Without detracting from his achievements, the philosophical and scientific context is important to acknowledge in order to understand why he was successful in altering the whole concept of circulation. Anatomical knowledge had leaped forward in the previous century with the publication of *De Humani Corpus Fabrica Libri Septum* in 1543 by the Flemish anatomist Andreas Vesalius (1514–64), in which he elucidated the anatomy of the heart and blood vessels. Harvey graduated from Padua in 1602 having studied under a former pupil of Vesalius, Hieronymus Fabricius (1537–1619), who had written on 'the little doors in the veins' in De Venarum Ostiolis of 1603, so Harvey is likely to have been aware of Vesalius' work. Hence, he may have known that Vesalius had exposed the fact that Galen had performed his dissections on the Barbary ape rather than human cadavers and that Vesalius had contested Galen's belief in a porous ventricular septum that his dissections failed to demonstrate.

A Spanish physician, Michael Servetus (c. 1511–53) had also queried the existence of ventricular pores and wrote in a theological treatise called *Christianismi Restitutio* (The Restoration of Christianty) of 1553 that blood must flow from one side of the heart to the other through the lungs. His book also criticised the notions of predestination and the Trinity and was therefore considered heretical by the Christian church. It was burnt together with its author so his insights did not reach a wider audience. These were dangerous times to challenge the Christian church's authority but a growing number of scholars were doing so in different fields of enquiry. Just as medicine had been arrested by rigid adherence to ancient authority, so too had astronomy. Nicolaus Copernicus (1473–1543) reluctantly published *De Revolutionibus Orbium Coelestium* [On the revolution of the celestial spheres] in 1543, in which he argued that the sun, not the earth, was the centre of the universe. Galileo Galilei (1564–1642), who had studied medicine, provided further evidence, with the aid of a telescope, for the Copernican system, for which he was put on trial and placed under house arrest. Galileo also realised that the pendulum, whose movement he compared to his own pulse, would be useful in recording time. His interest in mechanics and measurement influenced the evolution of medical thought.

A further reason why the time was right for a medical paradigm shift lay in philosophical reform. Francis Bacon (1561–1626), philosopher and statesman, advocated critical thought and an inductive method of reasoning based on experience. In his book *Novum Organum* [New method] (1620) he suggests that the four 'idols' – namely, accepted authority, popular opinion, legal bias and personal prejudice – should be abandoned. René Descartes' (1596–1650) assertion that the body was 'a machine made by the hand of God' (Discourse on the Method of Rightly Conducting One's Reason and Seeing the Truth in Sciences, 1637) was attractive to a new school of medical thought, which regarded the body as mechanical in nature. One particular advocate was Sanctorius Sanctorius (1561–1636) of Padua, where he was a professor after Harvey had left. He designed a number of measuring instruments including the 'pulsilogium' or pulse clock. A more accurate timing piece was designed in 1704 by Sir John Floyer of Lichfield (1649–1734), the physician's pulse watch, which ran for 1 minute.

Harvey adopted an experimental method that provided irrefutable evidence for his theory that the heart pumps blood and that blood circulates around the body. In a series of lectures to the Royal College of Physicians, he demonstrated that as the total volume of blood pumped from the left ventricle in 1 hour far exceeds that contained in the entire body, 'it is a matter of necessity that the blood perform a circuit, that it returns to whence it set out' (*De Mortu Cordis*, 1628 [On the motion of the heart and blood]). Like so many of his predecessors and contemporaries, he was nervous at how his revolutionary ideas would be received, which explains his dedication to the president of the Royal College written at the beginning of his 70-page monograph, *De Motu Cordis*:

> [T]he studious and good and true do not esteem it discreditable to desert error, though sanctioned by the highest antiquity, for they know full well that to err, to be deceived, is human . . . I would not charge with willful falsehood any one who was sincerely anxious for truth, nor lay it at any one's door as a crime that he had fallen into error. I avow myself the partisan of truth alone . . .

Indeed, the work did give rise to controversy but it won the day. Harvey had no visual evidence for capillaries, but these were later found by Malpighi, who was enabled by a microscope (*see* Chapter 5 in this section, 'From toy to tool: the microscope'). Nor did Harvey have an explanation for why the blood circulated. This was to come later in the wake of the following discoveries.

- Robert Boyle (1627–91) showed that air was essential to life and for combustion.
- Robert Hooke (1635–1703) showed that artificial respiration kept an experimental animal alive, so it was the air and not simply its movement that maintained life. The orthodoxy had been that the lungs cooled down the heart through their bellow action.
- Richard Lower (1631–91) repeated Hooke's experiment to show that dark blood travelling through the lungs regained its bright red colour when the animal received artificial respiration. He concluded that the entrance of fresh air was necessary to maintain life. He went on to perform the first transfusion from animal to animal.

- John Mayow (1643–79) described fully the mechanism of respiration and concluded 'some constituent of the air necessary to life enters into the blood in the act of breathing'. (*Tractatus quinque medicophisici*, 1774 [Medical Physical works])

The first tentative attempts at measuring blood pressure were made in the 1730s by Stephen Hales (1677–1761), a fellow of the Royal Society. He prepared an 11-inch-long glass tube, which he inserted into the arteries of a horse. His measurements, based on how far the blood moved up the glass, erroneously showed a large difference between pressures in the extremities and centrally. Almost a hundred years later in 1833, Jean Louis Marie Poiseuille (1797–1869) used a U-shaped tube containing mercury and with this was able to disprove Hales' findings. Not until 1896 was an accurate instrument designed that did not require skin incision; Scipione Riva-Rocci (1863–1937) created the prototype of today's instrument, using an inflatable band to which air was pumped until the pulse disappeared. Harvey Cushing (1869–1939), an American neurosurgeon, was impressed by this non-invasive method as a means of measuring vital signs.

> **Questions**: How did measuring blood pressure improve medical practice? What measurement was yet to be routinely recorded and who devised the technique for doing so?

Why is this relevant?

- We probably do not always appreciate how revolutionary a scientific approach was and how hard it was to question established dogma. Maintaining a critical and questioning approach to our work is still a challenge. This might be more of a problem in the future as clinicians come to rely increasingly on the new accepted 'dogma', the clinical guidelines. In contrast, those clinicians who want to make a judicious choice not to follow the guidelines are likely to be deterred by possible sanctions.
- Measuring blood pressure or the pulse involves simple and safe instruments that can be used in a variety of settings, including a person's home. So many investigative procedures of the modern day are complex, expensive and non-portable. Patients are often required to travel to a centralised location and undergo procedures that can be quite frightening and certainly alien to their experience. Are the disadvantages and costs always justified? Do clinicians today, because of medico-legal concerns, over-investigate?

Further reading

Wright T. *Circulation: William Harvey's revolutionary idea*. London: Chatto and Windus; 2012.

5

From toy to tool: the microscope

IT IS EASY FOR US NOW TO BE SOMEWHAT BLASÉ ABOUT HEADLINES championing new achievements in the power of microscopes: 'New microscope produces dazzling 3D movies of live cells' (Howard Hughes Medical Institute [website], 4 March 2011) but how exciting it must have been in the 1600s to discover a world of which the unaided eye was completely oblivious – a world of mountains, ravines and multitudinous swimming creatures. However, this new toy, the microscope, could only be put to serious use in the study of disease once it was possible to visualise specimens clearly and with good magnification. This took some time to happen.

The principle of the simple microscope and telescope was accidently discovered by spectacle makers Hans and Zacharias Janssen from Holland, sometime between 1590 and 1610. The microscope consisted of a short tube made of an opaque material with a lens at one end and a flat glass plate at the other, with the object to be observed placed at this end. The images were blurry and magnification may only have been nine-fold. By the 1660s, well-made microscopes were commonplace in Holland. A professor of physiology, Athanasius Kircher (1602–80), was the first to make a serious study of disease using a microscope. He examined the blood of plague victims and concluded that the objects he saw were minute living organisms; in fact, they were probably red blood corpuscles, since his microscope did not have the power to visualise microorganisms. Nonetheless, he correctly inferred that contagious diseases were conveyed by small organisms invisible to the human eye. It would be almost another 200 years before scientists who had access to considerably more sophisticated microscopes proved him right.

Question: Who were these scientists and what did they demonstrate?

The magnification power of microscopes was much improved by Dutch merchant Antonie van Leeuwenhoek (1632–1723), who spent his life in perfecting the simple microscope, which had only a single lens that could produce a 200-fold magnification. He made numerous observations, including of bacteria sourced from the white film of his own teeth, protozoa and spermatozoa, which he was the first to describe. The Royal Society of London published his work and made him a fellow.

Practising medicine: diagnostic methods

The first principle curator of the Royal Society was Robert Hooke (1635–1703), who published a book in 1665 based on his weekly microscopic demonstrations for the society called *Micrographia*. The book contains a description of a section of cork that he refers to as a 'cell' because the structural arrangement he saw reminded him of the rooms in which monks lived; this was the first time the word was used in such a context. His book had a major impact due to his skill as a draughtsman – his drawings caused great excitement. Hooke was also first to use a basic three-lens configuration in his microscopes.

Another pioneer of microscopy was Marcello Malpighi (1628–94), a professor at Bologna who identified the anastomosis between arterial and venous capillaries in 1661, thereby providing some of the proof for William Harvey's (1578–1657) explanation of circulation. Harvey had assumed the existence of small vessels between the arteries and veins to allow blood to circulate around the body but lacked the visual evidence. Sadly, Harvey had died 3 years before Malpighi's discovery (*see* the previous chapter in this section, 'The beat, beat, beat of the drum: the discovery of circulation and the tools to measure it').

Unfortunately, there were drawbacks to the microscope, which led to a diminution of interest in its medical and scientific potential during the eighteenth century. This was because of the problems of chromatic and spherical distortion. 'Chromatic distortion' occurs due to unequal bending of different colours in the light spectrum when passing through the lens, while 'spherical distortion' occurs due to unequal bending of light that hits different locations of the lens – both these processes result in blurring of the viewed specimen and the presence of a distorting halo around it. Errors were therefore common. It is possible that the myth of the 'homunculus' – the fully formed human in each sperm droplet – may have resulted from microscopic distortion (*see* Section 3, Chapter 3, '"The sperm of men is full of small children" and other early ideas about conception'). These problems were eventually addressed in 1830 by a wine merchant, Joseph Jackson Lister (1786–1869; father of Joseph Lister, who later championed antisepsis in the operating theatre). He discovered both how to realign the colours using a second lens of different shape and light-bending properties and the optimal distance that lenses needed to be set apart. In 1872, Ernst Abbe (1840–1905) worked out a mathematical formula, later to be known as the 'Abbe sine condition', which achieved maximum resolution. In other words, he discovered laws that govern the collection of light by the microscope's objective to maximise the sharpness of the image. This was the first time that microscopes could be built based on a precise mathematical formula rather than trial and error. Abbe and Carl Zeiss (1816–88) continued to perfect the microscope at their company Zeiss Opticals, thus the manufacturing of high-quality microscopes moved to Germany.

In the early twentieth century, Ernst Ruska (1906–88) developed the electron microscope, which uses electrons rather than light to 'illuminate', enabling visualisation of objects as small as atoms. These microscopes became commercially available from the Siemens company in 1939.

Why is this relevant?

- The microscope represented a significant medical breakthrough: it destroyed the concept of spontaneous generation and allowed identification of the microorganisms responsible for contagious disease. This led to effective diagnosis and then to disease prevention and treatment.
- The contemporary descendants of the humble microscope include the scanning probe microscope, which is able to explore the nano-universe and even manipulate molecules.

Further reading

Wilson C. *The Invisible World: early modern philosophy and the invention of the microscope.* Princeton, NY: Princeton University Press; 1997.

Section 7

Practising medicine: interventions and cures

1

The appeal of the miracle cure

DESPERATELY ILL PEOPLE ARE EXTREMELY VULNERABLE TO THE APPEAL of the 'miracle' cure, which allegedly offers a solution to a problem that conventional medicine cannot tackle. This tendency has manifested in different ways, but remains as familiar today as it was over 200 years ago.

The ready availability of 'patent' medicines was a feature of the marketplace in eighteenth-century England. There was no regulation of the ingredients for these mixtures, and no Trade Descriptions Act, so the claims of manufacturers did not have to be proven. The most popular labels included alcohol- and opiate-based concoctions that were to some extent addictive (as we may perceive with hindsight), but there was also brisk business to be done by anyone promising a cure for venereal disease. Newspaper advertisements referred allusively to 'stubborn' or 'obstinate' complaints, and gave full details of where people could buy the relevant pills, ointments and jollops.

Sexually transmitted diseases such as syphilis and gonorrhoea carried a threefold penalty for their sufferers: they may have provided embarrassing evidence of sexual infidelity or promiscuity, they could have proved exceedingly painful in the short term and they could eventually cause death. In the eighteenth century, the only active and apparently effective treatment for syphilis was mercury.

Question: How was mercury administered to patients – orally, anally or topically?

Mercury seemed to tackle the symptoms of syphilis, but it carried some dramatic and unpleasant side effects. It stimulated the production of saliva to a massive extent, such that mercury treatment became popularly known as being 'salivated' for the pox. Prolonged exposure to mercury caused people's teeth to fall out prematurely, and we can now appreciate that the properties of mercury would have had a lasting and deleterious effect on people's neurological functioning. In this context, any treatment promising to cure venereal diseases with discretion or that claimed patients might avoid the pain and obvious physical side effects of mercury, inevitably attracted hopeful customers. In a pre-antibiotic world, none of these supposed cures carried a realistic likelihood of successful treatment, but they certainly played on the hopes and fears of contemporary sufferers.

In the twenty-first century, cancer probably takes the prize for the disease invoking maximum dread. It has features of earlier, much feared maladies, such as the potential for sudden onset and acute pain, in addition to a relatively high chance of terminal diagnosis, despite modern chemical and radiotherapy treatments. Immunisation against cervical cancer, which was implemented in the British Isles for adolescent girls from 2008, was the first notable prophylactic measure to be used against any form of cancer.

'Miracle' cures for cancer have become a regular feature of the popular press in Britain. For example, in 2005 the *Daily Mirror* reported the case of a woman whose breast cancer appeared to have been entirely eradicated by recourse to mistletoe (J Disley, 'My breast cancer was cured by mistletoe', *Mirror News* [online], 24 December). She apparently rejected the surgical and chemotherapy options offered by the NHS and chose instead to inject herself with mistletoe among other herbal and relatively non-invasive treatments. The inclusion of the story on 24 December flags some of the newspaper's interest in the story; it was a 'good-news' item that coincidentally carried a seasonal theme, given the traditional use of mistletoe for Christmas decoration. The *British Medical Journal* responded to this and other similar stories a year later in December 2006, casting considerable doubt on the use of mistletoe, both because randomised clinical trials have yet to show that it can benefit cancer sufferers and because self-medication with mistletoe can promote the proliferation of some cancers (Ernst E. Mistletoe as a treatment for cancer. *British Medical Journal*. 23–30 December 2006: 1282).

Why is this relevant?

- The twin desires to prolong life and avoid pain remain key motivators and will prompt people who are otherwise sensible to try risky or unproven interventions.
- The management of patient expectations and the inculcation of realistic goals by medical practitioners have a long history of being frustrated and/or convoluted by the media.
- The picture is complicated by the demonstrable placebo effect exhibited by some treatments.
- The rise of homoeopathy and other alternative therapies since the early 1970s has occurred in part due to a dissatisfaction with mainstream medicine and because such treatment may additionally offer the desperate time to talk and hope.

2

Medical misdirection

NUMEROUS MEDICAL TREATMENTS HAVE BEEN TRIED IN THE PAST. Many were inspired by the prevailing model of health and illness held at the time. Others were discovered serendipitously and some were cynical attempts to deceive the public. This chapter focuses on just three interventions: bloodletting, electrical treatment and mesmerism. Their exponents were on the whole well-intentioned but they could not always guard against misuse and descent into quackery.

Bloodletting was a standard treatment for a variety of conditions from Hippocrates' (c. 460–c. 370 BC) time to at least the middle of the nineteenth century. It was a rational approach but misguided, as it was based on an erroneous model of illness. The humoral theory proposed four bodily constituents, namely blood, phlegm, black bile and yellow bile, which led to disease when out of balance. According to the influential Greek physician, Galen (129–c. 200 AD), most disease was due to *plethora*, an excess of one or more of the humours. Starving, vomiting, purging and bloodletting were the orthodox treatments used to rid the patient of this presumed excess. (*See* Section 6, Chapter 1, 'Early Greek and Roman contributions', for more on humoral theory.) Bloodletting was consistently advised by respected physicians in Europe and America for the next 1800 years. That is a long time, given that the bleeding was mostly ineffective or harmful and, at times, fatal.

Question 1: What developments occurred to discredit bloodletting as a standard treatment?

Medical debate was not on whether bloodletting was a useful intervention but on procedural details, such as from where the blood should be drawn, how often and how much. Over the centuries, there were a few sceptics such as Thomas Sydenham (1624–89), known latterly as the 'English Hippocrates', and a physician from Nottingham, England, Marshall Hall (1790–1857), who described the lancet as 'a minute instrument of mighty mischief' in his book *Diagnosis of Diseases* (1817). He produced guidelines for the 'rational employment' of bloodletting having accrued data on animals. In 1828, a French physician and pathologist, Pierre-Charles Alexandre Louis (1787–1872), using a statistical technique that he called the 'numerical method', concluded that bloodletting was ineffective for patients suffering from pneumonia and other feverish conditions. His insight met with resistance from many French physicians who, in the 1820s and 1830s, used 'copious bleeding', as advocated by the influential Parisian physician François Broussais (1772–1838). However, Louis' numerical method marked the beginning of a more objective medical approach to decisions on the efficacy of treatment; it was the forerunner of the clinical trial.

The techniques used for bleeding ranged from venesection and cupping to the use of leeches. Scarification was performed using a tool known as a 'scarifactor', a spring-loaded lancet attached to several blades. In cupping, the cups or small bulb-shaped containers made of glass or ceramic were heated to make a vacuum and used to dilate the superficial blood vessels, which were then lanced. Leeches were used where cupping glasses were not suitable, such as for the lips, vagina or haemorrhoid veins:

> Leeches are highly useful, and can be applied to the most delicate parts, as the eyes, gums, breasts, testicles etc where cupping can not be employed. It is sometimes a difficult matter however to get them to stick and when this happens it will be necessary . . . to smear them over with a little milk or fresh blood . . .
>
> R Thomas, *A Treatise on Domestic Medicine*, 1822

Once satiated, the leeches would drop off and could be reused by getting them to disgorge the blood with a sprinkle of vinegar. Leeches were especially popular in France, where the annual demand was about 3 million in the early nineteenth century, and this figure rose eight-fold during the 1830s.

Another popular medical treatment of the nineteenth century was that of therapeutic electricity. Alessandro Volta (1745–1827) invented the first battery at the end of 1799, and Michael Faraday (1791–1867) discovered the induction current in 1831, which was the first continuous electrical current. A spate of medical publications on the applications of electricity to practical medicine followed that increased interest among British medical practitioners. In 1836 Dr Golding Bird (1814–54) was put in charge of a new department at Guy's Hospital, London for treatment of patients by electricity and galvanism, which boasted its own 'electrical room'. He treated a range of conditions such as epilepsy, paralysis, chorea and even amenorrhoea and reported his findings based on case studies in a series of lectures, published in the Guy's Hospital Reports. He was not alone in his interest. Following the discovery of the vasomotor nerves, electric currents were used with increased confidence to treat migraine. In fact, Elizabeth Garrett Anderson (1836–1917), the first British female doctor, who paved the way for women to be accepted into medical school, wrote in her doctoral thesis *Sur la Migraine* [On migraine] that voltaic electricity was one of the most effective treatments.

Bird was an initial supporter of the Pulvermacher hydro-electric chain, which he thought would be convenient to treat patients with paralysis in their own home because of its portability. However, he soon distanced himself from its exponents' therapeutic claims, which extended to correcting impotency. The chain was constructed as a series of linked voltaic cells that could be worn around the waist and was able to impart electric shocks. Its 'clinical' application for impotency became so well known, that Gustave Flaubert (1821–80) referred to it in his book *Madame Bovary* (1856) through the character of Monsieur Homais, whom he describes as 'more bandaged than a Scythian'.

> **Question 2**: We may be amused at some of these treatments, but there has been renewed interest in the therapeutic uses of electricity in the twentieth and twenty-first centuries. For what conditions has it been revived?

A further treatment that became popular in the late eighteenth century was 'animal magnetism' or 'mesmerism'; the word 'animal' is derived from the Latin *animus*, which means soul. This intervention was proposed by a Viennese physician, Franz Mesmer (1734–1815), who rejected the four humours of humoral theory in favour of the presence of one vital and universal fluid that connected humans and animals to inanimate objects. Mesmer believed that this life 'energy' moved through the body freely but resulted in sickness when blocked. This concept is similar to the Chinese notion of 'chi' and is held by other vitalist doctrines often found in traditional medical practice. Mesmer believed that a human conductor of this energy, a 'magnetiser', was capable of healing through directing universal fluid towards a sick person. He initially used magnets to achieve this but later just his hands, which he passed over parts of the patient's body. Some aspects of mesmerism later developed into spiritualism and were incorporated into the theosophical movement. One particular medical exponent of mesmerism was Benjamin Rush (1746 or 45–1813), a Founding Father of the USA and influential physician who was also an advocate of copious bleeding. The Scottish physician and surgeon James Braid (1795–1860) was also a supporter initially but later rejected mesmerism for hypnotism, which he postulated was successful due to a 'peculiar physiological state of the brain and spinal cord' (Tinterow M. *Foundations of Hypnosis: from Mesmer to Freud*. Springfield: Charles C. Thomas: 1970. p. 320); today it has become a popular but controversial treatment.

While Mesmer was practising in Paris in 1784, a Royal Commission was set up to investigate whether there was any evidence for mesmerism and to interrogate the practice of one of Mesmer's disciples. It concluded that magnetic fluid did not exist and its apparent effects were due to the imagination of its subjects. Their report did not initially harm Mesmer's practice, although he was later driven out of Paris.

Why is this relevant?

- Medical interventions usually reflect prevailing theories of illness. When these are wrong, treatments are as well.
- The advent of modern epidemiology and the clinical trial, which emphasises

the importance of population rather than individual comparisons, has added objectivity and credibility to medical treatments.

● Even today, despite rigorous research and sophisticated analysis, new treatments may still be excessively praised before further experience of their use proves them less effective than first thought or even harmful.

Further reading

Bivins R. *Alternative Medicine? A history*. Oxford: Oxford University Press; 2007.

3

The rise of pharmacology: a story of prepared minds, money and serendipity

PHARMACY IS AN ANCIENT PURSUIT, WHICH ONLY BECAME INDUSTRIAL-ised in the mid-nineteenth century. Artificial synthesis of specific drugs could not occur until pharmaceutical chemistry had sufficiently progressed. The first step in this journey was to identify and isolate active therapeutic agents in natural drugs. This only became possible at the beginning of the nineteenth century, when a German pharmacist, Friedrich Sertürner (1783–1841), isolated the first ever alkaloid from a plant, which he named 'morphine' (after the Greek god of dreams, Morpheus), a naturally occurring chemical found in unripe seeds of the poppy.

The first medicinal drugs came from natural sources such as herbs, roots, fungi and trees. Several ancient civilisations developed a corpus of knowledge about the therapeutic benefits of these botanicals for specific medical complaints. For example, the first Chinese pharmacopoeia, *Bencao Jing* [The Divine Farmers Herb-Root Classic] is attributed to the Emperor Shennong who lived about 2700 BC. It contains a classification of medicinal plants and a guide to medical compounds. The Egyptian *Ebers Papyrus* (c. 1550 BC) refers to 700 drugs and methods of administration, such as: for asthma, a mixture of herbs should be heated on a brick so that the sufferer can inhale their fumes; to evacuate the belly: 'Cow's milk 1; grains 1; honey 1; mash, sift, cook; take in four portions'; and '[t]o remedy the bowels: Melilot, 1; dates, 1; cook in oil; anoint sick part'.

Greek pharmacy largely drew on both Egyptian and Asian therapeutic botanical knowledge. There is some suggestion that the Greek myths about the exploits of gods and heroes were a repository for this knowledge. An illustration of this is the story of Jason of the Argonauts, who on visiting the island of Colchis, known for its extensive magic and medicinal plants, returns with *Colchicum autumnale* (autumn crocus or meadow saffron), which the Arabs later discovered as useful for gout (*see* Section 5, Chapter 3, 'Broken bones and failing joints). Hippocrates' (c. 460–c. 370 BC) writings of the fifth century BC identify over 200 specific drugs as well as provide details about their administration. The first known illustrated herbal was produced in the first century BC by a botanist and physician named

Crateuas, which Pedanius Dioscorides (c. 40–90 AD) drew on to write *De Materia Medica* [Of medical material] in 60 AD. This compendium became a basic source of plant knowledge for 1500 years; among other remedies, mandrake and henbane are recommended as potent analgesics. Much of Greek and Roman scholarship was preserved by a Roman, Aulus Cornelius Celsus (c. 25–c. 50 BC), whose book *De Medicina* [Of medicine] of the first century BC also described Roman surgical procedures for cataracts, bladder stones and setting of fractures. This work was republished in 1478 at a time when no other Classical book on medicine was in print. Similarly, Paul of Aegina, who lived in the seventh century AD, provided an important legacy in his *Epitomes Iatrikes Biblio Hepta* [Medical compendium in seven books].

Greek and Roman medical learning would not have survived the fall of the Roman Empire but for Christian monks who transcribed many of the ancient works and the Arabian scholars who made the effort to translate them into Arabic. At this time, Islamic culture was progressive and eager to acquire Western medical learning in accordance with the Prophet's strictures: 'O servant of God, use medicine, because God hath not created pain without a remedy for it' (Abu Huraira. *Book of Bukhari*, volume 7 book 7, number 71).

Arabic medical understanding particularly contributed to medicine through observations on the use of drugs. Indeed, the word 'drug' is of Arabic origin, as are the words 'alcohol', 'alkali', 'syrup' and 'sugar'. The Arab pharmacopoeia included benzoin, camphor, saffron, myrrh, laudanum, senna and naphtha. Various chemical procedures were invented or refined by the Arabic people, such as distillation, evaporation, filtration and crystallisation. A flourishing medical school developed in Baghdad as well as a pharmacy. Several important medical works were written by Muslim physicians such as Rhazes (865–925 AD), whose book *al-Hawi* [The comprehensive book] was published in Latin in 1486 and Ibn Sina, or Avicenna (980–1037 AD), whose fifth book of *Al-Qanoon fi al-Tibb* [The canon of medicine] is entirely about the action of drugs and their preparation. *The Canon*, which firmly expounds Galenic doctrine, became the most authoritative text in the medieval universities until the late sixteenth century. These Arabic books made their way to Europe through Spain and southern Italy to the Salerno Medical School where Constantine the African (c. 1020–87 AD), a Tunisian physician, translated them into Latin in the eleventh century. Salerno also produced the *Regimen Sanitatis Salernitanum* [The Salernitan rule of health], which was written in verse. It became a popular self-help guide in the Middle Ages and provided advice on diet and drugs; the fact that it was written as a poem was probably intentional. This made it easier to remember and enabled it to be passed on orally by a largely illiterate population.

Western alchemy became a source of knowledge about chemical procedures throughout the Medieval and Renaissance periods. This discipline was based on Aristotelian philosophy and embraced mysticism and spirituality. Its main objective was to discover the philosopher's stone, which could turn base metals into gold and silver as well as produce an elixir of life. Paracelsus (1493–1541) was a physician and alchemist in the early sixteenth century who thought that chemicals could be used therapeutically. He believed that the purpose of alchemy was not to create gold but to discover and prepare substances with medicinal properties. This iatrochemical approach was an important precursor to modern pharmacology. Various natural philosophers such as Sir Isaac Newton (1642–1727) and Robert Boyle (1627–91) were also very interested in alchemy. In his book *The Sceptical Chymist* of 1661, Boyle argued that the so-called four (Aristotelian) elements are actually composed of 'corpuscles' (atoms), which are capable of organising themselves in groups to form chemical substances. He thus challenged the Aristotelian view (based on Empedocles) that just four elements – air, earth, fire and water – compose all matter (*see* Section 6, Chapter 1, 'Early Greek and Roman contributions').

Question 1: Boyle is often considered the father of chemistry. What is he remembered for?

Drug production became industrialised in the nineteenth century. There were various reasons for this:

- scientific advances in other emerging disciplines such as chemistry, physiology, microbiology and biochemistry; in chemistry, the discovery of alkaloids was a turning point since they facilitated isolation of the active constituents of other substances
- the success of the textile and dye industries, which explored whether the by-products of dye production could be useful by providing marketable drugs
- the American Civil War (1861–65), which led to a huge need for antiseptics and analgesics
- the discovery and isolation of active therapeutic agents in botanicals – such as morphine in 1804, quinine in 1820, atropine in 1833 and cocaine in 1860 – which led to attempts to synthesise natural products and to produce improved versions.

In the USA, a number of companies emerged, whose names are still well known. For example, Edward Robinson Squibb's (1819–1900) laboratory prospered when war broke out in 1861. It was responsible for developing a chemically pure form of ether and of chloroform that helped to improve the safety of anaesthetics. George Smith's company also benefited from the Civil War, expanding to become Smith, Kline and French. Following the war, other companies were established, such as Eli Lilly in 1876 and Merck in 1891, which was a subsidiary of a leading German chemical company.

In Europe, the chemical industry was thriving. Switzerland was the centre of trade in textiles and dyestuffs. Manufacturers there realised that dyes had antiseptic properties, which they were quick to market. Bayer was established as a dye maker in 1863 in Germany and soon moved into drug production. This switch occurred on discovering that some of the by-products of coal tar, such as derivatives of aniline and p-nitrophenol, had analgesic and antipyretic properties. At the turn of the twentieth century, Bayer produced the first blockbuster drug, which it called 'aspirin'.

In the second half of the nineteenth century, Germany dominated the drug production market. This changed during the First World War, when German subsidiaries and trademarks in the USA were seized, thereby allowing the American pharmaceutical industry to catch up; however, German drug manufacturing recovered between the wars under a vast conglomerate called IG Farben, which included Bayer among other large companies.

The inter-war years saw three significant discoveries, all of which were arguably serendipitous. Bayer thought that synthetic dyes may have specific antibacterial properties and appointed Gerhard Domagk (1895–1964) in 1927 to investigate, which he did methodically by experimenting on infected mice. Eventually, he discovered that the dye sulphonamidochrysoidine (marketed as Prontosil) was effective in killing bacteria. Following his publication in 1935, scientists at the Pasteur Institute in France found that the drug's therapeutic properties were due to another chemical to which the dye was linked – sulphonamide – rather than the actual dye. Sulphonamides were extensively used during the Second World War, since the other major antibiotic discovery, penicillin, was not produced in sufficient quantity to meet military needs until 1944.

Question 2: What other infections did sulphonamides help to cure?

The story of penicillin illustrates both the importance of chance events being noticed by a prepared mind and the potential for slippage between discovery and application (*see* Section 4, Chapter 8, 'Water as a historical force'). Alexander Fleming (1881–1955) had worked for many years on natural defences against wound infections and had identified the enzyme lysozyme, which is a component of the body's defence mechanism. On returning to his laboratory following a holiday, he noticed that a mould had appeared in a Petri dish and that it seemed that the mould had killed colonies of *Staphylococcus*. Although he published on penicillin in 1929, he did not pursue his discovery and his paper did not receive much interest. One reason Fleming may not have continued was the difficulty in extracting, purifying and stabilising penicillin. In 1940, two Oxford scientists, Howard Florey (1898–1968) and Sir Ernst Chain (1906–79), achieved this. Through Florey's professional contacts in the USA, he was able to expedite penicillin production there on a large scale in late 1941. Fleming, Florey and Chain were each awarded the Nobel Prize for Medicine in 1945.

Question 3: What was serendipitous about the discovery of insulin?

Two events cast a dark shadow over the story of pharmaceutical chemistry: experimentation during the Second World War and the effects of thalidomide.

A former Auschwitz prisoner testified:

There was a large ward of tuberculars on block 20. The Bayer Company sent medications in unmarked and unnamed ampoules. The tuberculars were injected with this. These unfortunate people were never killed in the gas chambers. One only had to wait for them to die, which did not take long ... 150 Jewish women that had been bought from the camp attendant by Bayer, ... served for experiments with unknown hormonal preparations.

www4.dr-rath-foundation.org (accessed 6 May 2013)

At the Nuremberg Trials, an SS physician, Dr Waldemar Hoven, testified that these experiments were undertaken by the big pharmaceutical conglomerate IG Farben: '[T]hey only took place in the interests of IG, which strived ... to determine the effectiveness of the preparations ... It was not IG's intent to make any of this public'. (www4.dr-rath-foundation.org)

However, the end of Second World War did not bring an end to the rapacity of some pharmaceutical companies. Thalidomide, which was marketed in 46 countries in the late 1950s and early 1960s as an anti-emetic for pregnant women with morning sickness, led to around 10 000 babies being born with a variety of deformities; hence, in 2012:

German drug firm issues first apology to thalidomide victims

...

Freddie Astbury, president of Thalidomide UK, described the company's apology as a 'disgrace' and called on the company to pay out compensation.

The 52-year-old from Liverpool was born without arms or legs after his mother took the drug.

'I'm gobsmacked,' he said. 'For years, (Gruenenthal) have insisted they never did anything wrong and refused to talk to us.'

Mr Astbury said he and other British survivors had received some money over the years from a trust set up by [T]halidomide's UK distributor but that Gruenenthal had never agreed to settle.

B Henderson, *The Telegraph* [online], 1 September 2012

Question 4: What were the consequences to the pharmaceutical industry of this tragedy?

Why is this relevant?

- Plants were the main source of medicine until the nineteenth century and continue to serve as the basis of many pharmaceutical drugs.
- The initial discoveries of active therapeutic agents were indebted to chance rather than design. The interests of capitalist pharmaceutical industries combined with progress in pharmaceutical chemistry led to a therapeutic revolution, which tentatively began at the turn of the twentieth century and reached is apogee in the 1940s, 1950s and 1960s.

- Greater ethical strictures and strict regulation of drug testing before licensing are relatively recent developments in human history. There are certainly benefits to the public from this but also arguably some disadvantages.

Further reading

Lax E. *The Mould in Dr Florey's Coat: the remarkable true story of the penicillin miracle*. London: Abacus; 2005.
Le Fanu J. *The Rise and Fall of Modern Medicine*. London: Abacus; 2011.

4

From party games to pain control: the story of anaesthesia

NO DOUBT PEOPLE HAVE ALWAYS TRIED TO CONTROL PAIN. HARD evidence of this exists from at least the third millennium BC thanks to the discovery of opium poppy seeds in Mesopotamia. This was the location of the Sumerian civilisation and translations of their cuneiform scripts found on stone tablets suggest the use of poppy seed to relieve pain. Most civilisations have developed analgesic recipes of varying efficacy composed of mixtures of ingredients such as alcohol, opium, scopolamine, hemp and cannabis. During the Han Dynasty, a highly regarded Chinese surgeon, Hua Tuo (c. late 2nd–early 3rd century AD), used a herbal concoction called 'mafeisan' to anaesthetise his patients, which probably comprised a boiled mixture of cannabis and other ingredients. In the Western world, *Mandragora* (mandrake) was used in 1298 AD by another prominent surgeon, Theodoric of Lucca (1205–98 AD), for its ability to provide surgical relief; he soaked a sponge in a mixture of opium and mandrake and applied it to the patient's face to inhale. This plant was associated with some sinister beliefs and referred to by William Shakespeare in *Romeo and Juliet*:

> And shrieks like mandrakes torn out of the earth,
> That living mortals hearing them, run mad.

Act 4, Scene 3, lines 50–51

We know now that mandrake's active ingredients include scopolamine, hyoscyamine and atropine, which account for its ability to produce skeletal muscle paralysis and anaesthesia. However, the future of anaesthetic agents was not to remain with orally ingested substances.

Nitrous oxide was isolated by Joseph Priestley (1733–1804), who wrote up his research on gases in 1774. In 1798, Thomas Beddoes (1760–1808) founded the Pneumatic Institute in Bristol to research the therapeutic potential of gases. He collaborated with James Watt (1736–1819), of steam engine fame, to design equipment that could deliver Priestley's gases. Humphry Davy (1778–1829) was appointed director of the institute and conducted several experiments using nitrous oxide, which he discovered relieved him of toothache and made him giggle. Tantalisingly close to altering medical practice and patient experience, he observed that it might be of use surgically but made no attempt to apply his insight. He called it 'laughing gas', which may have done it no favours in being accepted by the medical profession, especially since it was used as an entertainment for the public, notably by Samuel Colt (1814–62) who toured the USA to raise finances to put his new revolver into production.

It fell to an empathic dentist, Horace Wells (1815–48) to rediscover the potential of this inhalable gas in relieving pain and who, following a number of experiments on his own patients, decided to publicise his discovery. Sadly, his demonstration at Massachusetts General Hospital in 1845 was unsuccessful because he had under-dosed the patient who suddenly cried out in pain. Wells experienced considerable public humiliation from this event, which may have led him to become addicted to chloroform. Under its influence, he threw sulphuric acid at two women and was subsequently confined to an asylum where he hung himself. One year later, Well's collaborator and apprentice William TG Morton (1819–68) successfully removed an ulcerated tooth from patient Eben Frost using ether and shortly afterwards demonstrated its use at Massachusetts General Hospital. On 16 October 1846, he painlessly removed a tumour from a patient's jaw using a simple apparatus to apply the ether vapour. This impressed the audience, particularly a rather sceptical chair, Dr John Collins Warren (1778–1856), founder of the *New England Journal of Medicine*, who was moved to conclude 'This is no Humbug' (Fenster JM. *Ether Day*. New York: Harper Collins; 2001). Morton was quick to patent his 'discovery' and tried to hide the active anaesthetic ingredient by calling his product 'Letheon' but the genie was out of the bottle. By November 1846, Henry Bigelow, a junior surgeon at the same Massachusetts hospital had published an account of the demonstration (Bigelow HJ. Insensibility during surgical operations induced by inhalations. *Boston Med Surg. Journal* 1846; 35: 309–17) and news quickly spread across the Atlantic.

Ether's anaesthetic properties had actually been known for some time. The alchemist and physician Paracelsus (1493–1541) observed in 1525 that chickens exposed to ether 'undergo prolonged sleep and wake unharmed'(www.general-anaesthesia.com (accessed 6 May 2013)). However, by the 1800s, like nitrous oxide, its main use was in entertaining the paying public at events that came to be known as 'Ether Frolics'. Medical students used the vapour recreationally and ether drinking became an acceptable alternative to alcohol for abstainers.

One of these public shows was attended by an American physician, Crawford Long (1815–78), who noted that participants had no recall of experiencing minor injuries on stage while taking ether. Although he experimented with ether using one of his medical students, James Venables, from whom he had removed a neck cyst in 1842, he did not publish his findings until 1849 because he was uncertain whether the induced anaesthesia was a placebo effect. It should be said that Venables had readily agreed to be a guinea pig because of his fear of pain. In 1846, the Scottish surgeon Robert Liston (1794–1847) performed the first operation in Europe with ether, remarking that 'this Yankee dodge beats mesmerism hollow' (www.historyofsurgery.co.uk (accessed 6 May 2013)) (on mesmerism, *see* Chapter 2 in this section, 'Medical misdirection'), but the medical profession was slow to adopt it. This was mainly because of its side effects, such as coughing and lung congestion, and the difficulty in assessing correct dosage. John Snow (1813–58) addressed the latter problem through a series of experiments in which he showed that concentration could be determined by temperature. Thus, he was able to develop a safe administration technique.

Attitudes towards pain control varied particularly with regard to labour. 'Unto the woman he said "I will greatly multiply thy sorrow and thy conception: in sorrow thou shalt bring forth children"' (Genesis 3:16). This quote illustrates the Christian church's disapprobation of pain control during labour and although its disapproval may have been overstated, it is often cited as one reason for reluctance in adopting chloroform. Sir James Simpson (1811–70) was a great advocate of pain control and went so far as to retranslate the Old Testament from the Hebrew to show that that there was no religious reason why women should not be given pain relief during labour and that pain was not a necessary accompaniment to giving birth. As accoucheur to Queen Victoria, he made sure she received his pamphlets based on his paper in *The Lancet* in 1847, titled 'On a new anaesthetic agent more efficient than sulphuric ether'. She decided that Simpson would attend the delivery of her eighth child rather than her regular obstetricians. On 7 April 1853, Simpson poured some chloroform on a handkerchief and she breathed from this. Her endorsement, particularly as head of the Church of England, removed much of the stigma associated with pain relief in childbirth: 'Dr Simpson gave that blessed chloroform and the effect was soothing, quieting and delightful beyond measure.'

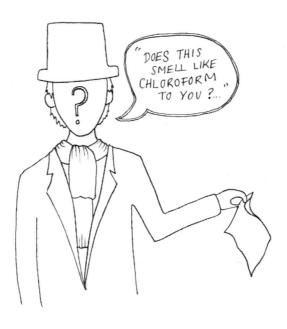

However, medical critics of pain control remained unconvinced. Some of their concerns were reasonable, others based on false premises and prejudice. One professor of obstetrics at Jefferson Medical College, Charles Meigs (1792–1869), believed that labour pain was a sign of the 'life-force'. This sentiment reflected a common medical belief that pain was a good sign because it kept the body alive. Given that Meigs once revealed a degree of chauvinism with a remark about the size of an obstetric patient's head ('almost too small for intellect and just big enough for love'), his disinterest in pain control may not be surprising.

> **Question**: What do think were the reasonable medical concerns about the new anaesthetics?

Simpson, like many other doctors of the time, often experimented on himself and his friends. Convinced that chloroform was safe, he would throw dinner parties at which the guests inhaled chloroform; it is said that he would kiss his female guests as they passed out. Morton paid people in the street to try his ether and coerced his assistants to take it. Long's first operation using ether was on a medical student.

> **Discussion point**: Self-experimentation has a long history in the medical world. Without it many advances would have been at best delayed. Can it ever be justified in the present?

Chloroform soon developed a dark side, being linked with robberies and rapes in which victims asserted they had been suddenly overcome by being forced to inhale the vapour. Its reputation as a surgical aid, however, appears not to have diminished, despite the continued social risks. In 1994, a doctor from Liverpool was convicted for abducting and raping a young woman using chloroform. More recently, in 2008, the death of 3-year-old Caylee Marie Anthony in Orlando, Florida, was alleged to be due to the administration of chloroform.

Why is this relevant?
- The advent of reliable and safe anaesthetics allowed the surgical speciality to develop operative procedures that previously were quite impossible given the imperative of keeping the duration of operations to a minimum.
- Anaesthesia must be considered one of the greatest medical advances in history in terms of relieving human suffering and, in conjunction with the aseptic technique, saving lives.
- Ethical standards in the nineteenth century allowed for human experimentation that would be quite unacceptable today.
- Attitudes towards pain control appear to have significantly altered; however, it is only recently that more attention has been given to ameliorating the pain of terminal illness and chronic disease.

Further reading

Snow SJ. *Operations without Pain: the practice and science of anaesthesia in Victorian Britain.* Basingstoke and New York, NY: Palgrave Macmillan; 2006.

Stratmann L. *Chloroform: the quest for oblivion.* Gloucestershire: Sutton Publishing Ltd; 2003.

www.historyofsurgery.co.uk

www.churchinhistory.org

www.general-anaesthesia.com

www.histansoc.org.uk

5

Transplantation

A RECENT HEADLINE IN THE GUARDIAN PROCLAIMED: 'UK'S OLDEST living kidney donor, 83, gives his organ to a stranger' (Press Association, 17 May 2012). Apart from the difficulty in some developed countries of procuring organs, people today take it for granted that advances in medicine allow for failing organs to be easily replaced. However, until just 40 years ago, this proposition was arguably tantamount to suggesting the creation of a chimera.

In the *Odyssey*, Homer (c. eighth or seventh century BC) describes the 'chimera' as a creature with a goat's body, lion's head and dragon's tail. Although a living organism composed from another or several other living beings was a wild fancy, modifications of this fancy regularly emerge across various eras and cultures. For example, according to Taoist teachings, the Chinese physician Pien Ch'iao (c. 700 BC) performed a heart operation between two men under anaesthetic to correct their respective imbalance of 'qi' (life force) and *zhi* (will). There are several references in the New Testament of Christian saints restoring body parts to their owners after trauma, but an attempted replacement of a whole leg with one cut from a cadaver by Saints Cosmos and Damian marks a shift of thinking.

More credible accounts of early transplantation describe the practice of skin grafting from the second century AD. This expertise was based on the works of the famous Indian surgeon Sushruta (c. 750 BC), who had pioneered skin transplantation for rhinoplasty, probably because the practice of cutting noses was a common punishment for criminal offences. His writings were lost, although fortunately not before an Arabic translation was made in the eighth century AD. This found its way some centuries later to Europe, where, in Italy, Gasparo Tagliacozzi of Bologna (1545–99 AD) became familiar with his techniques; in 1596 he reported on his own technique of using a skin flap from the upper arm to repair an injured nose. Some of these operations were undertaken for cosmetic reasons – it was common practice for a slave with a handsome nose to be required to donate it to their master or mistress! – but these operations did not usually work: 'When the date of nock was out, off dropt the sympathetic snout', wrote the English satirical poet Samuel Butler (1612–80) in *Hudibras* (1663–78).

Although experience taught surgeons that it was almost impossible to transplant organs successfully from another body, there were exceptions. John Hunter (1728–93), surgeon and anatomist, performed a successful xenograft when he

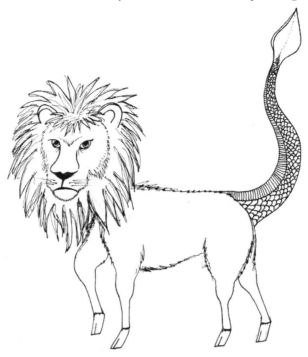

transplanted teeth into the well-vascularised comb of a cock. He went on to transplant teeth between people, discovering that the chances of success were best when the donor tooth was as fresh as possible; however, other sources suggest that donated teeth never really bonded with the recipient's gums for long.

Skin grafting to cover granulating surfaces was performed in the nineteenth century but these grafts did not usually last long either. One exception was that of an allogenic skin transplant that Winston Churchill supplied. He described it as merely 'a piece of skin and some flesh' donated to a fellow soldier during the Boer War; however, by the beginning of the twentieth century, the most successfully transplanted organ was that of the cornea, with the first such transplant performed on a human in 1905 by Czech ophthalmologist Eduard Zirm (1863–1944).

The reasons for the high failure rate of organ transplantation were not understood at the turn of the twentieth century and continued to elude medical practitioners for several more decades. No less than 500 publications on the subject had been published by 1910, with the overall conclusion being that heterotransplants invariably failed, autografts were almost always successful and graft success was more likely when donor and recipient had a close blood relationship. Nonetheless, substantive progress was checked for almost another 50 years.

The first successful renal transplant occurred between identical twins Richard and Ronald Herrick and was performed by Joseph Murray (1919–2012) in Boston in 1954. However, subsequent transplantations between close relatives led to the appalling statistic of just five of 91 patients surviving for 1 year post-transplant.

> **Question 1**: Why would it be difficult to continue operating with such a high failure rate in contemporary medical practice?

There were three challenges to overcome before transplantation could hope to be more successful and these required interdisciplinary collaboration:
1. understanding of how the immune system fights transplantation
2. the development of surgical techniques to anastomose small blood vessels
3. the discovery of an effective immunosuppressant.

The following individuals, all Nobel Prize winners, performed lead roles in addressing these challenges.
- Sir Peter Medawar (1915–87), a British immunologist and Nobel Prize winner for his work on acquired immunological tolerance, worked out that the theoretical basis for transplant rejection was cell mediated.
- Joseph Murray developed a surgical technique based on that devised by French surgeon Alexis Carrel (1873–1944), who had treated an assassinated president in 1894. Carrel realised that the internal bleeding caused by the knife wound could have been stopped if he had been able to anastamose the severed blood vessels. From 1902, he performed several transplants on dogs to perfect a method of achieving this.
- George Hitchings (1905–98) and Gertrude Elion (1918–99) were involved in a research programme to find a chemical that could prevent cancer cells from multiplying and discovered 6-Mercaptopurine. A haematologist, William Dameshek (1900–69), started to consider using it to block replication of immune-system cells.

Unfortunately, even with the benefits of a second version of 6-Mercaptopurine, called 'azathioprine', reports in 1963 at a Human Kidney Transplant conference held in Washington were overall very disappointing. However, there was one exception – surgeon Thomas Starzl's (1926–) post-operative management slightly differed to that of his colleagues. He very carefully monitored his patients and, at the first sign of organ rejection, administered high doses of steroids to defuse rejection. In 1 year, he performed 33 renal transplants. Twenty-seven of the 33 patients remained alive with functioning kidneys; 15 of these patients were still alive almost 25 years later. Starzl went on to perform the first successful liver transplant in 1967. In the same year, Christiaan Barnard (1922–2001) performed a successful heart transplant.

> **Question 2**: What other advances helped to improve the survival rate among transplant patients?

The scandal referred to in the headline 'Alder Hey pathologist struck off' (D Batty and agencies, *The Guardian*, 20 June 2005) involved a pathologist who had taken children's organs without parental consent from 1988 to 1994, and eventually led to the Human Tissue Act 2004; this implemented much stronger regulations in regard to the removal, storage and use of human tissue. However, public concern about the medical use of corpses is not new.

One of the biggest scandals in Victorian Britain was that of William Burke and William Hare, who supplied Scottish anatomist Robert Knox (1791–1862) with bodies for dissection (required for Knox's successful anatomy school in Edinburgh). Burke and Hare did not snatch bodies from among those recently interred in graves but instead killed to maintain a supply of fresh and therefore lucrative cadavers. Anatomists were desperate for fresh dead bodies to dissect because, prior to the Anatomy Act 1832, only the bodies of executed murderers could be legally dissected, so they were in short supply. The act stopped the practice of the 'resurrectionists' by allowing for access to those dead from the workhouses who had not been claimed by their relatives within six weeks of death. This greatly increased the supply for anatomy departments. However, the act was much distrusted in poorer communities, as people feared that bodies would be sold quickly by parish authorities to the anatomical schools to meet their costs of care prior to death. Neither did the public believe that all the body parts would be returned intact for burial following dissection; this was unacceptable on religious grounds for those who believed that a dissected body could not rise from the grave whole on the Day of Judgement. Protests occurred – one such protest took place at Cambridge in 1832, when a dissection theatre was vandalised to stop a man being dissected.

Why is this relevant?

- A shortage of teaching material in the early nineteenth century led to illegal means of procuring corpses. An apparent shortage of research material led to a pathologist at Alder Hey Children's Hospital in Liverpool retaining children's organs without consent. Both scandals led to new legislation and distrust in the medical establishment.
- Current public expectation of what medicine can achieve through organ transplantation is high but thwarted by the lack of donors. There are 7000 people on the kidney waiting list in Britain but one person dies every day while awaiting a suitable organ. Attempts at increasing organ supply, such as by a system of presumed consent, need to be aware of both historical distrust of the medical establishment and religious sensitivities.

Further reading

Bates AW. *The Anatomy of Robert Knox: murder, mad science and medical regulation.* Eastbourne and Portland, OR: Sussex Academic Press; 2010.

Moore W. *The Knife Man: blood, bodysnatching, and the birth of modern surgery.* New York, NY: Doubleday; 2006.

6

Cutting for the stone: the hazards of surgery

SURGICAL INTERVENTION IS ONE OF THE OLDEST MEDICAL TREATMENTS known to humanity. There is evidence that trephining the skull to treat depressed skull fractures or to release demon spirits, dates back to 10 000 BC. Most surgical procedures in ancient times were minor and the approach conservative, as apparent from descriptions in Egyptian papyri of c. 1550 BC of removal of abscesses and small tumours. One exception was the attempt to remodel noses in Hindu India, where the practice of lithotomy also occurred. Hippocrates' (c. 460–c. 370 BC) was very cautious about performing this operation preferring to leave it to itinerant 'cutters' or 'incisors': 'I will not cut for stone, even for the patient in whom the disease is manifest. I will leave this operation to be performed by specialists' (*Hippocratic Oath*).

The term 'lithotomy' was coined by Ammonius of Alexandria (third century AD) in about 200 BC, a Greek surgeon who performed the operation by breaking up the bladder stones to make removal easier. The first clear description of this procedure in Western literature was given by Aulus Cornelius Celsus (25 BC–50 AD) in *De Medicina* [Of medicine] (20 AD). The procedure required just two instruments, a knife and a hook, and was thereby called the 'lesser' operation. It involved a midline perineal incision, which carried deeply into the bladder. The offending stone was pushed forward by a finger in the rectum and, with the help of a bladder full of urine, gushed out. The drawbacks were that it was only advisable in boys aged 9 to 14 years and 50% of those who underwent the operation died! Even so, it continued to be employed until the Renaissance, when the 'Marion' or 'greater' operation was introduced.

The greater operation was characterised by an incision made on the left side of the perineum and used more instruments than the lesser operation, including a grooved staff to guide other instruments up the urethra having first dilated it. Dilation often tore the prostate and bladder neck leading to haemorrhage; a special pair of forceps with blades attached was used to grasp and crush the stone. If the patient survived, he could anticipate side effects such as a fistula, incontinence and erectile dysfunction. One flamboyant lithotomist, the monk Jacques de Beaulieu (1651–1714), adopted and popularised this lateral method.

At first, his fatalities were impressively high, probably because his anatomical knowledge was limited, although he later corrected this deficiency and went on to perform some 5000 operations in Europe.

Samuel Pepys (1633–1703) was operated on for a stone by Thomas Hollyer of St Thomas' Hospital on 26 March 1658. So pleased was he at the operation's success, he celebrated its anniversary every year, despite his consequent sterility. Quite clearly, the pain of having bladder stones drove men to risk their lives and endure acute pain to have them removed.

> Dec 3, 1659
> Being this morning (for observacion sake) at the Jewish Synagogue in London I heared many lamentacions made by Portugall Jewes for ye death of Ferdinando ye Merchant, who was lately cutt (by the same hand wth my selfe) of ye Stone.
>
> Samuel Pepys, *Diary*

Question 1: Bladder stones are a less common complaint in the twentieth century. Why?

By the eighteenth century, lateral lithotomy was at its height of popularity due to the improvements William Cheselden (1668–1752) had made to the operation. He kept bleeding to a minimum by the use of ligatures and cut rather than tore tissues. His mortality rate was comparatively low, side effects far fewer and healing time only 1 to 3 months. Cheselden had also tried a different operation called 'suprapubic cystotomy', which he published on in 1723 in *A Treatise on the High Operation for the Stone*; however, this approach had been introduced by John Douglas (d. 1743) in 1719, so Cheselden gave it up because he did not want to be accused of plagiarism. In any case, the method did not catch on, even though it was a simpler operation, because of the risks of rupturing the peritoneum and causing peritonitis.

Cheselden was a popular surgeon known for his quickness in the operating theatre. He was responsible for leading a movement to separate the London surgeons from the Company of Barber-Surgeons. The Surgeons' Guild and Company of Barbers had been amalgamated in 1540 under Henry VIII, although their functions were separated; barbers were employed in bloodletting, teeth extraction and cutting hair. In 1745, the separated Surgeons' Company became a trade guild, which at the end of the eighteenth century transformed into the Royal College of Surgeons. During the nineteenth century, professional standards were raised, and admission to the college was restricted to those who could pass an examination on having completed 6 years of study at a recognised London teaching hospital. London became the leading surgical centre in Europe between 1840 and 1870, partly because there were so many hospitals in London and the population comparatively large.

Lithotomy continued to become a safer operation in the nineteenth century.

This was in part due to a French surgeon, Jean Civiale (1792–1867), who founded the first urology department in the Necker Hospital in Paris and invented the lithotrite in 1832. The introduction of antiseptic techniques was also a major factor in reducing mortality.

Question 2: How did antiseptic surgery come about?

Before the mid-nineteenth century, lithotomy was the most commonly performed operative procedure after amputation. Antisepsis, followed by asepsis, and anaesthesia transformed surgical practice (*see* Chapter 4 in this section, 'From party games to pain control: the early story of anaesthesia'). The next technical discovery to have a highly significant impact on surgery was that of the X-ray.

Why is this relevant?

- Significant advances in surgery could only occur once other disciplines had made discoveries: anaesthesia in dentistry, germ theory in chemistry, X-rays in physics. Medical advances continue to be dependent on interdisciplinary collaboration.
- Closed minds and prejudice can delay beneficial innovation.

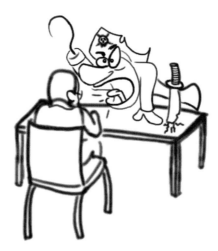

What?! Are you telling me that I cut my hand off for this hook for nothing because you have improved the techniques of lithotomy now?!

Further reading

Carter KC, Carter BR. *Childbed Fever: a scientific biography of Ignaz Semmelweis.* Brunswick, NJ: Transactions; 2005.
Ellis H. *History of Bladder Stone.* Oxford: Blackwell Science; 1969.

Section 8

Healers and health carers

1

From spicer to pharmacist

THE EARLY DEVELOPMENT OF ANY PROFESSION IS OFTEN CHARAC-
terised by boundary disputes between groups of people claiming the same
competencies. To meet this challenge, a fledging profession will seek to con-
solidate its identity with new measures such as the introduction of harder entry
criteria, higher educational demands, regulation and monitoring of standards.
Institutions spring up or evolve to support and ensure these changes occur, and
new legislation is frequently enacted to support enforcement. The rise of the
pharmaceutical profession both in Europe and the USA provides a good example
of this journey.

In the previous section, Chapter 3, 'The rise of pharmacology: a story of
prepared minds, money and serendipity', traced the development of pharmacology and the pharmaceutical industry from ancient times, when pharmacopoeia
were first written, to the twentieth century. These texts were repositories for a
collective knowledge of the therapeutic botanicals amalgamated over centuries
and contained recipes for compounds that required skill and care to prepare.
Medieval monastic orders developed those skills, since they were often the main
providers of healthcare to the poor. Not only did they run hospitals but also
pharmacy shops supported by the monastery's herb garden. One of the first of
these pharmacies in Europe was attached to the famous cathedral of Florence,
St Maria Novella.

In thirteenth-century England, a number of different people could supply
medical drugs, including spice merchants, grocers and physicians as well as
apothecaries. Apothecaries were members of the grocers' guild, the Worshipful
Company of Grocers, which included pepperers and spicers. The former were
the wholesalers and the latter the retailers of drugs; the terms 'apothecary' and
'spicer' soon became interchangeable. Over time, the apothecaries felt they
deserved the same status as physicians, taking the view that they were performing much the same role in providing medical advice, albeit to the working and
peasant classes. Further, they wanted the right to prescribe drugs. Unsurprisingly,
they were not impressed when Henry VIII empowered the College of Physicians
in 1540 to 'search, view and see the apothecary wares, drugs and stuff'. Their
response was to show their worth by requesting to be examined not just for their
knowledge about drugs but also about medical practice. Although this did not

happen immediately, by 1607 they were recognised as a special body within the grocer's company and by 1617 they had separated into a new organisation, the Worshipful Society of Apothecaries of London. As an independent body, they were able to make entry to their society dependent on successful completion of an examination. The grocers became solely traders, since they were no longer allowed to make medicines or to advise on their use.

By the mid-eighteenth century, the apothecary had assumed the skills and roles that we would now recognise as those of a GP and had really become part of the medical profession. Thanks to the Rose case at the beginning of that century (Royal College of Physicians v. Rose, 1704), they enjoyed the same prescribing rights as physicians. Like physicians, they examined, diagnosed, prescribed for and treated patients, although usually these were from the poor or working class. Indeed, Adam Smith (1723–90), an influential moral philosopher, acknowledged the apothecary 'as the physician of the poor in all cases, and of the rich when the danger or distress is not very great' (*Wealth of Nations*. 1776). However, unlike the physicians, they were not allowed to charge for their services; their income solely rested on dispensing medicines. As early as 1682, the apothecaries' society founded a commercial company which produced pharmaceutical products and won the exclusive right to supply the British navy. By the eighteenth century, the company had become the main supplier for the East India Company, and as a result, accrued considerable wealth.

The apothecaries were keen to secure a monopoly for compounding and dispensing drugs, which both druggists and chemists were still able to do; chemists were particularly skilled at making medical substances using distillation techniques or heat. The apothecaries criticised the chemists and druggists, accusing them of selling impure foreign drugs and leaving out costly ingredients of compounds to maximise their income. There were counter-accusations from the druggists that apothecaries colluded with physicians and were guilty of ignorant practice and lack of self-regulation. By the 1800s, the leading London apothecaries had formed the General Pharmaceutical Association, which petitioned parliament for the establishment of an examining body and regulation not just of apothecaries but surgeon-apothecaries (since, by this time, many apothecaries sat the College of Surgeons' exam), midwives and dispensing chemists. Further, the association demanded a monopoly on the sale of all medicinal preparations and preparing of physicians' prescriptions. The chemists successfully saw off this attempt to restrict their autonomy by arguing that they were more experienced in preparing medicines than the apothecaries, therefore should not be under their control. They also quickly proceeded to improve their image by introducing standards, monitoring and regulation. The ensuing Apothecaries Act 1815 supported the chemists and druggists by directing that apothecaries should not have a monopoly on making medicines.

Thereafter, the professional development of chemists into what we now recognise as the profession of pharmacy was encouraged by a number of socio-economic factors, one of which was an emerging class of people, especially in the industrial north of England, desirous of medical attention. Apothecaries could meet this demand but only with the help of the chemists, who had the time and expertise to prepare medical compounds. A further boost to the profession was the development of the first schools of pharmacy in the second half of the nineteenth century, such as in Brighton in 1858 and Manchester in 1883.

In contrast to England, physicians and pharmacists belonged to the same guild in thirteenth-century Florence. This guild had significant responsibilities and powers, such as examination of all its candidates, organisation of the placements of pharmacists, dictation of the price of drugs and supervision of production and sale of medicinal herbs. In the Kingdom of the Two Sicilies, pharmacy was heavily regulated by Frederick II (1194–1250), one of the most powerful holy Roman emperors of medieval times. He issued a number of decrees between 1231 and 1240 that resulted in pharmacy becoming recognised as a specialist area distinct from medicine and practice was monitored, prices for remedies were fixed and the number of pharmacies limited. Professionalisation similarly developed rapidly in Germany and France, where educational demands made of apprentice pharmacists in the guilds were high. Pharmacy as a university discipline with dedicated professors was also established much sooner in these countries than in England, leading to research and status.

The development of a pharmacy profession in the USA did not occur until the turn of the twentieth century, although the physician and Founding Father of the USA Benjamin Franklin (1706–90), had created an apothecary post at the Pennsylvania General Hospital in 1751 because he thought that drug dispensing should be a specialist occupation. There were no guilds in America and almost anyone could sell drugs which were mostly available in drug stores owned by druggists rather than physicians. 'Patent' medicines – secret formula remedies advertised directly to the public, often as dramatic 'medicine shows', for all kinds of ailments – proliferated. One example was that of Dr Thomas' Eclectic Oil, which claimed to cure:

> toothache in 5 minutes,
> earache in 2 minutes,
> backache in 2 hours,
> lameness in 2 days,
> coughs in 20 minutes,
> hoarseness in 1 hour,
> colds in 24 hours,
> sore throat in 12 hours,
> deafness in 2 days,
> pain by burn in 5 minutes,
> pain of scald in 5 minutes.

Pharmacists and physicians became concerned about such claims and the influx of adulterated foreign drugs. A Drug Importation Act passed in 1848 proved unsuccessful in guaranteeing the standards of foreign drugs, due to a lack of training of inspectors and the imprecise nature of the accepted pharmacopeia. It was clear that the success of any legislation would be dependent on the professionalisation of pharmacists. In response, a number of colleges of pharmacy were established in various cities over the second half of the nineteenth century to set standards and monitor their members. By the end of the century, the American Association of Pharmacists had produced a template for legislative practice for the use of all states. The template framed the pharmacist as a distinct specialist who could not be a merchant or storekeeper. A regulatory board was required to examine, register and enforce a code of conduct. In 1906, against considerable vested interest (the annual revenue was over US$80 million by then for 'patent' medicines), the Pure Food and Drug Act was passed. This act is significant for various reasons, not least of which was the government's assumption of responsibility to maintain minimum safe standards of food and drugs sold to the public.

In 1937, 107 people died having taken an elixir of sulphonamide that contained the toxic solvent diethylene. This event highlighted the need to establish drug safety before marketing. The following year, the Federal Food, Drug, and Cosmetics Act was passed in the USA, which made provision for this.

> **Question**: A further tragic scandal occurred in the early 1960s. What was this and what was the legislative response?

Why is this relevant?

- The process of professionalisation is a complicated and at times lengthy one. For it to occur satisfactorily, various elements are required, including: establishment of high standards of education during training, entry to the profession only on completion of an examination, monitoring of subsequent practice, licensing and registration. Additionally, professional practitioners are expected to abide by a code of ethical behaviour. This is meant to safeguard the public and ensure that a professional will behave with integrity. In exchange, historically, there has been a tacit understanding that professionals are people who deserve respect.

- A number of other practical measures must occur to establish a body as a professional one. These include development of professional organisations that set and monitor standards, educational departments and journals to disseminate knowledge. Legislation is also needed to give authority to professional organisations to carry out their role, such as registration and licensing.

- Today, there are significant concerns among many contemporary health professionals that their professional status is being eroded due to resentment of elitism, increasing risk adversity and over-regulation. They fear that as they are de-professionalised, professional attitudes and goodwill may disappear.

- Stronger drug regulation has led to much longer testing programs of new drugs and higher costs. Concerns are expressed that this is at the cost of development of less commercially viable drugs, the proliferation of 'me, too' drugs that are of no proven additional benefit, aggressive marketing, high drug pricing and very long delays before drugs are available to the public.

- Just as in the past there were significant concerns about the purity of drugs sold to the public, today we also worry about standards of pharmaceuticals produced in foreign countries or sold over the Internet.

Further reading

Anderson A. *Snake Oil, Hustlers and Hambones: the American medicine show*. Jefferson, NC: McFarland; 2004.

Loudon I. *Medical Care and the General Practitioner.1750–1850*. Oxford: OUP; 1986.

Diminishing Nightingale: an alternative history of nursing

FLORENCE NIGHTINGALE (1820–1910) WAS ONE OF THE MOST FAMOUS women in Victorian England. She became a national heroine at the time of the Crimean War, and when she fell ill while abroad in 1855, the nation raised a fund in her name. The money collected, a staggering £44 000, was devoted to supporting training for 'lady' nurses and the rest, as they say, is history.

> **Question**: By how much was the mortality rate at Scutari Hospital, Istanbul, reduced in the 6 months after the arrival of Nightingale and her group of 38 nurses? Have a guess, then look up the answer.

Yet Nightingale's personal role in securing better training to produce higher-skilled nurses is questionable, because the cause she adopted had already been established before her actions in Istanbul. St John's House, an Anglican sister-hood founded in London in 1848 and also devoted to nursing, offered training and employment to working-class nurses. The establishment aimed to raise the character and reputation of nurses generally, by improving their working and living conditions. The stereotypical nurse in 1848 was a woman who was either so exhausted by her cleaning duties that she could not deliver medical support to doctors (by following their instructions and monitoring patient well-being) or who was feckless and immoral (because she left the ward without permission, drank alcohol while on duty or took perquisites from patients). St John's House sought to provide a decent income and respectable lodgings to sober, hard-working and reliable women. The trainees were taught to expect night as well as daytime shifts (long a bone of contention in hospitals, in which rivalries and tensions arose between the day staff and the night-time nurses). Importantly for the women involved, they were not expected to clean or undertake laundry, leaving them freer (and more alert) to respond to patient or medical requirements.

Crucially for the place of St John's House in the history of nursing, the sisterhood was asked to take over full responsibility for nursing at King's College Hospital in 1856. This was a highly successful move; so successful, in fact, that medical practitioners associated with the hospital arguably came to regret the arrival of women from St John's – they proved too independently minded for some of the doctors. Even so, the St John's experiment provided a model for others to follow, some time before the first of Nightingale's 'lady' nurses began training at St Thomas' Hospital in 1860.

Nightingale's personal role in managing her fund was minimal. After her return from the Crimea she threw herself into a new arena by becoming heavily involved with a Royal Commission into the army medical service. Further, she fell ill with a complaint (retro-diagnosis offers brucellosis as one possibility) and remained an invalid for the remainder of her life. She became an indefatigable writer, but her priorities after the war can be summarised as the reform of military medicine first; then the overhaul of colonial medicine, particularly in India; and sanitary reform in Britain in third place (of which nursing was only one component).

Further, the quantitative impact of the first Nightingale trainees was minimal in the short term. The women were technically contracted to train for a year and to serve as a hospital nurse for at least 5 years thereafter, being paid a wage throughout their 6-year contract. Of the first 'probationers', as they were called, four were hastily dismissed as unsuitable, while only four from the first intake were still in post after 2 years. A slow accumulation of women who completed the training and remained in nursing gradually had some effect, but the influence of the Nightingale scheme was far out of proportion to its recruitment.

Nightingale remained very influential, but her interventions in the field of nursing arguably restricted the professional and intellectual progress of the women involved (regardless of whether they had been trained by her fund). For example, the Royal British Nurses' Association (founded 1887) had the goals of statutory nurse registration and a measure of theoretical scientific education for the women, but it met with forceful opposition from both Nightingale personally and the fund more generally. The Nightingale Fund was opposed on the grounds that nursing was not the same as medicine, and should not aspire to similar structures as those enjoyed by medicine such as registration. The fund's administrators may also have been irritated by the British Nurses' Association's premise that registration would be predicated on 3 years of training (so would exclude the fund's trainees).

Therefore, the Nightingale name and the fund that bore it were much more important to nursing status, reform and professionalisation than Florence Nightingale was herself. Voices of doubt and deprecation have tended to focus on elevating the role of other individual women, such as Mary Seacole (1805–81; another woman actively nursing in the Crimea) or Sister Dora Pattison (1832–78; who worked in Walsall 1865–78 and was idolised following her early death). There is a case to be made, however, for the role of societal forces beyond the influence of specific actors, such as changing medical demands on nurses (particularly after the development of anaesthetics and antisepsis), the political appetite for employment reform and women's increasing confidence in public campaigns.

Why is this relevant?

- It is historically relevant to distinguish between the significance retrospectively attributed to Nightingale's influence and the level of her personal involvement with (and time for) nursing reform after her return to England in 1856.
- Nurses struggled to be regarded as honest and reliable employees at a time when doctors had already achieved statutory reform and regulation – a disparity that continues to influence the tenor of relations between doctors and nurses today.
- A *British Medical Journal* article of 1880 argued for nurses' 'blind obedience' to practitioners, in a context in which all London hospitals had training schools under the direction of a matron (Nurses and Doctors. *British Medical Journal.* 17 January 1880: 97–8). This suggests that the level of nurses' independence, autonomy and responsibility has been a matter of debate since nursing first aspired to professional status and shows no signs of being concluded. In February 2012, BBC News reported fears that nurse training had become too academic and a call for nurses to be 'compassionate as well as clever', which succeeded in irritating a number of medical groups (if for different reasons; see www.bbc.co.uk/news reported 29 February 2012).

Further reading

Baly ME. *Florence Nightingale and the Nursing Legacy.* London: Croom Helm; 1986.

Bostridge M. *Florence Nightingale: the woman and her legend.* London: Viking; 2008.

3

The origins of physiotherapy

PHYSICAL TREATMENTS SUCH AS MASSAGE, MANUAL THERAPY AND hydrotherapy were advocated by Hippocrates (c. 460–c. 370 BC) in the fifth century BC. When the speciality of orthopaedics began to develop in the eighteenth century (*see* Section 5, Chapter 3, 'Broken bones and failing joints'), a bicycle-like machine was designed by Frances Lowndes in 1796 to exercise all joints and muscles, called a 'gymnasticon'. However, the serious origins of modern physiotherapy as a speciality can be traced to the Royal Central Institute for Gymnastics founded by Pehr Henrik Ling (1776–1839) in Stockholm in 1813. The aims of the institute were to provide massage, manipulation and exercise for the sick. The idea of establishing an institute came to him after observing that taking daily exercise benefited his old joint injuries; at the time, he was a fencing instructor at Uppsala University. He decided to learn more about anatomy and physiology through attending courses and subsequently developed a system of medical gymnastics, which later became known as the 'Swedish massage system'. The system used techniques that resemble those used in Chinese massage, which he may have learned about through a Chinese friend who taught him about the martial arts. Initially, Ling's treatments were met with criticism from the medical establishment, but professional recognition came in 1831 when he was elected to the Swedish General Medical Association. His son and two former pupils carried on the speciality of medical gymnastics so successfully that the institute became officially recognised by the Swedish health authorities in 1887.

An important part of professionalism for any health discipline is that high standards of propriety are adhered to by health practitioners during a health transaction, particularly when it involves touching the patient. It is hardly surprising then, that the following debate prompted a brisk response:

The Alleged Massage Scandals
MR. S. SMITH (Flintshire) I beg to ask the Secretary of State for the Home Department whether his attention has been drawn to a statement made in The British Medical Journal that 'massage shops' are in many cases used for improper purposes; whether this subject has attracted the attention of the police …?

House of Commons Debates, 23 July 1894, vol. 27, cols 663–4

As a result of this apparent scandal, a number of nurses in Britain established the Society of Trained Masseuses in 1894, which set examinations and educational standards, inspected training schools and embraced diverse treatments such as hydrotherapy and electrotherapy. In 1900, the society incorporated specialists in remedial gymnastics.

There were two major catalysts to the development of the speciality during the early decades of the twentieth century: war and the polio epidemics. Ever since the medical speciality of orthopaedics evolved from the mid-eighteenth century, massage and remedial exercise had been used as an adjunct to more invasive therapy. During the First World War, American surgeons started to employ women with a background in physical education, called 'reconstruction aides' to restore function in injured soldiers. One of them, Mary McMillan (1880–1959), established the American Women's Physical Therapeutic Association (later renamed the American Physiotherapy Association) in 1921 and a journal for the dissemination of knowledge and experience. Another practitioner also helped the profession to grow – an Australian with extensive experience of injured soldiers, Elisabeth Kenny (1886–1952), who challenged orthodox approaches with her protocol of early mobilisation, muscular pain relief and a good relationship with patients.

The first major outbreak of polio was in 1916. In New York alone there were 8900 cases reported, of which 27% died. Although a very small percentage experienced acute paralysis, the majority of those did not recover full muscle strength. Several prominent and wealthy people contracted the disease, for polio was not only a disease of the poor. In 1921, Franklin D Roosevelt (1882–1945), who was then 39 years old and president of the USA, contracted polio, which produced paraplegia. His interest in alternative treatments led him to buy a spa at Warm Springs, Georgia, which became a centre for research and offered extensive hydrotherapy programmes with exercise. In 1937, he founded the National Foundation for Infantile Paralysis, which, together with the American Physiotherapy Association, raised significant funds to support research and increase the number of physiotherapists.

Question: Why is polio not a major health concern today in the Western world?

In 1920 in Britain, a Royal Charter was awarded to the Massage and Medical Gymnasts Society, which changed its name to the Chartered Society of Physiotherapists in 1944. Meanwhile, physiotherapy was becoming established in other countries. New Zealand, for example, set up its first school of physiotherapy in 1913, as did the USA in 1914, at the Walter Reed Army Hospital in Washington, DC.

Why is this relevant?

- Clinical practice often puts practitioners into much closer physical contact with patients than patients experience in everyday social encounters. Both parties need to be clear of the rules governing their behaviour and patients need to feel safe and be able to trust their practitioner. All health disciplines have strict codes of conduct, which are conveyed at a formative stage of training, and severe sanctions for infringements. Concerns about actions being misinterpreted have led particularly male practitioners examining women to require a chaperone. Although this is standard practice in the NHS, this is not always so in the private sector.

- Physiotherapy is the fourth largest healthcare profession in the UK. According to The Chartered Society of Physiotherapy, between 2000 and 2010 there was a 48% rise in full-time equivalent physiotherapists, but the demand continues to rise, especially with a growing older population. Only 60% of chartered physiotherapists work in the NHS, where there have been cuts to services in recent years.

Further reading

Young P. A short history of The Chartered Society of Physiotherapy. *Physiotherapy*. 1969; **55**(7): 271–8.

www.csp.org.uk

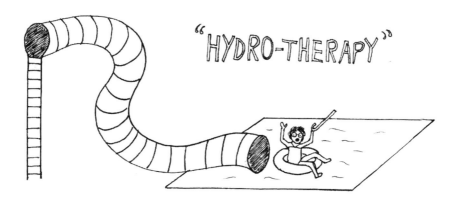

4

The shifting sands of health management

IN EARLY CIVILISATIONS, RELIGION AND MEDICINE WENT HAND IN hand. Priests provided places of healing in many cultures. In medieval Europe, hospitals were run by monastic orders. They served a dual function: the provision of accommodation for pilgrims and the care of the sick. This is illustrated by the etymological derivation of the word 'hospital', which arose from the Latin for guest, *hospes*. In England and Wales, the dissolution of the monasteries disrupted this system.

Diverse institutions gradually emerged to provide the services that monasteries had previously provided for sick poor and elderly. Significant legislation was passed, the Poor Laws of 1598 and 1601, which conferred a duty of care on parishes to support those sick who 'belonged' to their locality. The two London hospitals of St Thomas' and St Bart's were joined by philanthropic testamentary foundations such as Guy's Hospital and private subscription hospitals that developed across the British provinces. After 1834, workhouses with infirmaries provided a basic level of institutional cover. Arguably, these infirmaries constituted an embryonic national health service in providing free care to beneficiaries; workhouse hospitals certainly formed the backbone of the built facilities later transferred to the NHS.

The forms of administration of these institutions were as diverse as the institutions themselves. Community health service provision followed a similar but even more variable path, although private provision remained dominant. In Britain, the GP developed (*see* Chapter 1 in this section, 'From spicer to pharmacist'). His services were purchased and sometimes the purchaser might be a group of potential patients acting together in the form of a friendly society. There was very little administrative overview for this diverse system of provision and no clear rationale to develop one, given the fierce independence of some charities and most private practitioners.

In due course, the system became strained and reform became inevitable. Partly due to the successful experience of the Emergency Medical Service during Second World War and partly due to Labour Party ideology, the British NHS was established in 1948. Almost all hospitals (charity and workhouse) were taken over by the NHS and their staff became state employees, although senior doctors retained the right to private practice. GPs, dentists, pharmacists and opticians remained small businessmen and women, who contracted their services to the NHS. Local government continued to provide some community health services, although the bulk of their health provision, such as municipal hospitals and mental health services, was absorbed into the NHS. The Ministry of Health, headed by a cabinet minister, ran a tripartite service of:

- hospitals, through regional hospital boards and teaching hospitals
- independent health practitioners, such as GPs, dentists, opticians and pharmacists, through the Executive Councils
- community health services, through local health authorities and local Medical Officers of Health.

Individual hospitals were frequently administered simply by a hospital secretary, matron and medical superintendent.

Since then, however, managers in the health service have come to play a key role in the efficient delivery of healthcare. Their roles and numbers have increased significantly since the NHS was introduced. One of the main drivers for reorganisation was that of rising health costs; this, coupled with concerns regarding lack of clear lines of accountability, led to various reports advocating organisational change. One of the first was that of 1962 from the British Medical Association entitled *Report of the Medical Services Committee*, which concluded that area boards with adequate medical representation and a medical chief officer should replace the tripartite system. It also recommended that acute general hospitals should care for the long-term ill. Then, in 1967, the King's Fund and an Institute of Hospital Administrators' working party recommended that a general manager should have overall responsibility for each hospital and be supported by medical and nursing directors, a director of finance and statistical services and a director of general services. In the same year, the Ministry of Health published the *First Report of the Joint Working Party on the Organisation of Medical Work in Hospitals* (also known as the *Cogwheel Report*), which advocated the creation of clinical divisions to ensure efficient use of resources and the involvement of clinicians in management. In the event, the first major reorganisation of the NHS did not occur until the NHS Reorganisation Act 1973. Fourteen regional health authorities (RHAs), to which 90 area health authorities (AHAs) were accountable, replaced the tripartite system; each AHA was to have a chair appointed by the secretary of state and non-executive members appointed by the RHA and local authority. Area teams were created, each with an administrator, nurse, public health doctor and finance officer. GPs remained independent contractors. A further key development in the 1960s arose as a result of the *Report of the Committee on Senior Nursing Staff* (known as the *Salmon Report*) of 1967. The aim of the report was to increase the profile of the nursing profession in hospital management and to create a new nursing structure under a chief nursing officer. An alternative career pathway was now open to nurses.

Both political and medical dissatisfaction with the 1974 reorganisation led to another with the Health Services Act 1980, which set up 192 district health authorities (DHAs) to devolve management to smaller units of care. The 1980s witnessed two more major changes. First, Prime Minister Margaret Thatcher invited the Chair of the supermarket chain, Sainsbury, to head an inquiry into the health service. The inquiry party consisted of just four people and drew on consultations but no formal evidence. The *Community Care: agenda for action*, or *Griffiths Report*, of 1983, concluded that the health service lacked a coherent system of management and processes to evaluate its performance against normal business criteria. It recommended that the Department of Health and Social Security 'should rigorously prune many of its existing activities' and that general managers should be introduced and clinical doctors encouraged to become more involved in local management. Further, it wanted to see 'consensus management' – the orthodox management style until then – replaced by a top-down one of direction.

The second major change was the introduction of an internal market model. In this model, purchasers (GPs) and providers (mostly hospital services) were separated and GPs allowed to be the fund holders of their own budgets. This change was driven by a market economy ideology that promised to keep health-care funding competitive and low. New Labour, under Prime Minister Tony Blair, continued to support this approach from its election in 1997, albeit with a stronger emphasis on partnership and driven by performance. In the meantime, the Health Authorities Act 1995 brought in another reorganisation: RHAs were abolished and replaced with just eight regional offices. The DHAs and family health service authorities were merged. Devolution occurred in Wales, Scotland and Northern Ireland, such that these separate jurisdictions became responsible for their own health services; this resulted in increasingly diverse systems of health-service delivery across the UK.

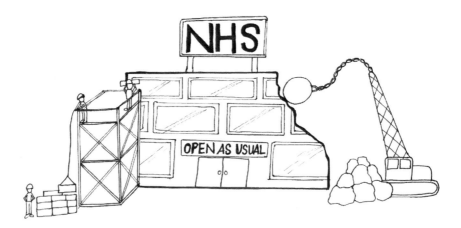

In England in 1999, GP fund holders were replaced with primary care groups. The NICE and Commissions for Health Improvement (known as Care Quality

Commissions in 2012) were established to monitor quality, governance and financial management. Blair pledged to raise NHS spending to match the European Union average and the government poured in investment, but many performance targets and standards for annual assessment were also set up. More administrators and project managers were required to meet the growing demand for information. Additionally, New Labour was committed to new public management to reform public-sector services. Gordon Brown, as chancellor of the exchequer, introduced Public Sector Agreements, which linked funding to targets for improving services, thereby influencing which health outcomes should be prioritised. Private-sector organisations were brought into the NHS as sources of funding through private finance initiatives and as private providers of independent treatment centres and some NHS walk-in centres.

In 2010, a new coalition government of Conservatives and Liberal Democrats came into power having pledged no further NHS reform; however, the realities of a serious national economic situation, rapid and demographically driven health-service inflation and the ideological attachment of some within the Conservative Party to the private sector, came together, resulting in the new Health and Social Care Bill. This abolished the Strategic Health Authorities and Primary Care Trusts and gave commissioning consortia, heavily influenced by GPs, the majority of the NHS budget for the health service, albeit under the supervision of a new NHS management board. At the time of writing, the consequences of this further reorganisation are unclear.

Question 1: What has been the consequence of the establishment of the NHS in the UK?

Question 2: What has been the consequence of central government increasingly seeking to micro-manage the NHS?

Why is this relevant?

- The rise of managerialism in the NHS was a phenomenon familiar to numerous sectors across the final quarter of the twentieth century and the first decade of the twenty-first. In this regard, has the NHS been at the forefront of change in the British context?
- The institutions and management of the NHS have been an inherently political (i.e. party-political) issue since its foundation and show no sign of shedding this attribute.
- Nigel Lawson (one of Gordon Brown's predecessors as chancellor of the exchequer) likened the NHS to the British national religion. If his assumption remains correct, any future reorganisations will inevitably be seen by the public as threats to a beloved national institution.

Further reading

Gorsky M. The British National Health Service 1948–2008: a review of the historiography. *Social History of Medicine*. 2008; **21**(3): 437–60.

Answers

Section 1: Emergency!

Chapter 1: Heroic patients

Q1: Why was Barnard not in attendance on Washkansky?

A: Barnard left his home in Cape Town soon after the operation, arguably to foster his incipient celebrity status. He was interviewed, photographed and generally feted around the world and used his fame quite blatantly to enjoy the fruits of a jet-set lifestyle (including multiple sexual conquests; he eventually divorced, and remarried a much younger woman). His medical renown was certainly secured by his being the first to transplant and reanimate a new heart in situ, but his long-term reputation as a professional suffered as a result of his active courting of admiration (that in justice belonged partly to Darvall and Washkansky). Compare Barnard's reputation with that of Norman Shumway (1923–2006) to compare their legacies as 'heroes'.

Q2: Who were Joe Burnside and Peter Everett?

A: Joe Burnside (1930–2008) became the longest-living heart transplant survivor in Britain. He received a new heart as one of the first patients at Papworth Hospital in 1980. Peter Everett (1962–80) was his donor. Everett was only 18 years old when he died from a brain haemorrhage, but he had already offered himself as an organ donor and had discussed the possibility of donating his kidneys in the event of his death. He had no anticipation of early death, since he was a regular competitor in athletic events. His mother therefore offered his heart as well.

Chapter 2: War wounds and amputees

Q1: Aside from physical suffering, what in particular did Burney find emotionally distressing about the operation?

A: Burney was affected by a variety of feelings, clustering around family and the imposition of medical authority. First, she was compelled to retain her composure while finding a pretext for her husband to be away from home on the day of the operation, as she wanted to spare him the direct evidence of her pain. She only had part of a day to anticipate the surgery but found the time spent waiting for her doctors interminable. When her medical team arrived, her initial reaction was one of affront at the number of people in her house apparently uninvited. Burney considered herself as much horrified by the visible preparations for her mutilation as by the prospect of pain and resisted some of her doctors' injunctions. Finally, she regretted the absence or early death of her sisters who might have provided moral support during such an ordeal.

Q2: How did her French doctors react to the procedure?

A: They were visibly nervous and somewhat upset, according to Burney's account.

Since she understandably screamed continuously while conscious, they clearly had to battle the contradictory pressures of removing the tumour entirely and the impulse to stop being the cause of immediate pain.

Chapter 3: Road traffic accidents: from horse carriages to motor vehicles

Q1: When did this legislation occur?

A: Legislation was passed on drink-driving in 1967 (Road Safety Act 1967), on seatbelt wearing in 1981 (Seatbelt Act 1981) and on handheld mobile phones and driving in 2003 (The Road Vehicles [Construction and Use] [Amendment] [No. 4] Regulations 2003).

Q2: What form of transport in Britain causes a disproportionate number of road traffic accidents?

A: Although only 1% of vehicle traffic is accounted for by motorcycles, 21% of road traffic accidents involve motor cyclists, who therefore have the highest mortality rate of any road user.

Chapter 4: Accidents in the workplace

Q1: What effects did these injuries have on families?

A: They deprived households of key earners and imposed additional costs for treatment or care at the same time. For further reflections on this topic, *see* Section 4, Chapter 2, 'Health and livelihood'.

Q2: What did the Health and Safety at Work Act etc. 1974 do?

A: It laid down general principles for protecting the workforce and allowed for specific requirements such as the disposal of hazardous products.

Chapter 5: Primary care begins at home

Q: How would the use of ground ivy in the treatment of coughs and mild lung complaints be regarded in the present day – as harmful, futile, remotely helpful or actively advisable?

A: One component of ground ivy, rosmarinic acid, is deployed in some modern medicines for its anti-viral properties. Rosmarinic acid occurs in other plants, so it is not exclusively found in ivy, but its presence there, combined with modern chemical understandings of its properties, would make the use of ivy in coughs and lung complaints potentially helpful.

Chapter 6: Fatality, the Coroner's Court and medical responsibility

Q: What organisations exist in the twenty-first century to support and advise medical professionals accused of negligence?

A: The Medical Defence Union was established in 1885, initially to assist doctors in meeting legal fees when they were sued, but, from 1924, it also indemnified practitioners for the full costs of compensation awarded against them. The Medical Protection Society was established in 1892 and the Medical and Dental Defence Union of Scotland followed in 1902. These societies have all survived to the present day and provide insurance cover to doctors worldwide.

Chapter 7: The history of resuscitation in England

Q: Can you find examples of some of the more outlandish methods for bringing people back to life?

A: Methods were varied, but they included tickling the back of the throat with a feather and inflating the patient with tobacco smoke via the rectum.

Chapter 8: From war to shell shock to post-traumatic stress disorder

Q1: What diagnostic symptoms of PTSD can you identify in this speech?

A: Kate describes her husband's sleep disturbed by nightmares of battles. The fact that he also 'starts so often' is probably a manifestation of hyper arousal. His decline in appetite, interest, pleasure and libido may be a result of a secondary depressive illness; affective changes are common in PTSD.

Q2: There were a number of other pioneers of medical psychology and psychotherapeutic approaches. Who were these people and where did they practice?

A: The psychologists were Charles Samuel Myers (1873–1946) consultant psychologist to the British forces in France, William McDoughall (1871–1938), former pupil of WH Rivers, and William Brown (1881–1952) who worked at Craiglockart hospital until 1919. Myers was responsible for persuading the military authorities to set up four advanced neurological centres behind enemy lines to deal with shell shock casualties. The idea was to enable early treatment and return to the battlefield. Due to his influence, the term 'shell shock' was officially dropped and replaced with the acronym 'NYDN' meaning 'Not yet diagnosed? Nervous'. Ironically, it was Myers who had first introduced the term 'shell shock'. The pioneering doctors were Richard G Rows (fl 1914–18), who worked at Maghull, Merseyside, England, and C Stanford Read (fl 1914–18), who worked at Netley, Hampshire, England, where courses in the psychotherapeutic technique of abreaction were given for army doctors.

Section 2: The pleasures of life: food, drink, drugs and sex

Chapter 1: The medical uses and abuses of tobacco

Q: The first lawsuits were brought against tobacco companies in 1954; why did it take so long for any the plaintiffs in these sorts of cases to achieve success? What did Adolf Hitler have to do with it?

A: Anti-smoking campaigns in the post-1945 period were hampered by the fact that the most outspoken government opposition to smoking to date had been voiced by Nazi Germany (where Hitler had been personally engaged in the movement).

Chapter 2: Sweet teeth: the history of sugar consumption

Q: How might sets of false teeth have been manufactured? What range of materials was available prior to the advent of modern plastics and chemical industries?

A: Teeth were most frequently replaced by other teeth – sets removed from cadavers and mounted in a frame or literally transplanted into the gum from living 'donors'; however, fabricated teeth might be devised using bone, wood or (for the wealthy customer) porcelain. Transplanted teeth did not always 'take', becoming discoloured and smelly. There was also a contemporary suspicion that they harboured disease.

Chapter 4: Friend or foe? Substance use

Q1: What is current Chinese government policy towards drug addicts?

A: According to Section 7, Article 347 of Criminal Law of the People's Republic of China:

> Whoever smuggles, traffics in, transports or manufactures narcotic drugs, and commits any of the following acts shall be sentenced to fixed-term imprisonment of fifteen years, life imprisonment or death, and concurrently be sentenced to confiscation of property...

In 2012, China abolished almost all of its death penalty sentences for offences.

Q2: What other explanatory models of addiction became popular in the second half of the nineteenth century?

A: There was significant debate about whether addiction was caused by moral weakness or a constitutional predisposition, with predisposing and precipitating factors. The latter model bracketed addiction with other conditions such as criminality, insanity and homosexuality, all of which came to be regarded as inheritable and presumed to progressively worsen as they were passed on through generations. This hereditary theory was called 'degenerationism' and provided a theoretical basis for the eugenics movement.

Q3: What were the consequences of the increase in heroin usage in the 1960s?

A: In 1965, the Interdepartmental Committee on Drug Addiction published its report (*The Brain Report*) proposing that only licensed doctors could prescribe heroin and cocaine, treatment centres for addicts be established and there be a system of notification to the Home Office. It also reaffirmed the view of the Rolleston Committee that addiction was a medical and psychiatric problem and not a matter to be dealt with solely by the criminal justice system.

Chapter 5: Before vitamins: the elusive ingredient

Q: Why might the improving health of the British navy and marine forces in the late eighteenth century have made a dramatic difference to the nation?

A: The period 1793–1815 was one of recurrent warfare in Europe, with Britain and France the main opponents. The British navy was vital to the military objectives of resisting invasion at home and defeating French forces abroad. Two naval victories in particular, at Aboukir Bay, Egypt, in 1798 and Trafalgar, west of Cape Trafalgar, Spain, in 1805, were important for shoring up the military effort and British morale. The latter became iconic partly owing to the death of Admiral Nelson from a sniper's bullet in the course of battle, but Nelson did not secure his victory alone. He famously signalled at Trafalgar 'England expects that every man will do his duty' (Schom A. *Trafalgar: countdown to battle, 1803–1805*. Oxford: Oxford University Press; 1992. p. 320). Of course, the ability of his men to act dutifully and effectively was substantially determined by their relative freedom from scurvy.

Chapter 6: Green sickness and other anaemias

Q: What made the pathology of sickle-cell anaemia particularly novel?

A: Sickle-cell disease was the first discovered 'molecular disease'. These diseases result from proteins with abnormal chemical structures.

Chapter 7: The 'single body' and changing understandings of sexuality

Q: Using Internet dictionaries of English phrases, research current thoughts about the origin of the saying 'lie back and think of England'. What is the most popular explanation of this expression epitomising female passivity? Which one do you think is right?

A: The first known published usage of the phrase is attributed to Alice, Lady Hillingdon (1857–1940) in one of her diary entries of 1912. However, it seems unlikely that the diary was the origin of the expression. Therefore, it was either in common use by 1912 or it was popularised by other means. There is no firm evidence for it originating with Queen Victoria, although a number of websites suggest this provenance.

Section 3: The facts of life: women, health and medicine

Chapter 1: 'On the blob' and other menstrual euphemisms

Q: What terms have you heard in use to refer to menstruation? Is this a question that you could ask your mother, grandmother or other female relations without embarrassment in the interests of historical research?

A: Clearly, everyone who reads this book will answer this question slightly differently. It is worth remembering that sanitary products were not advertised on television at all until the 1980s in Britain, and exponents of 'alternative' comedy in the same decade were the first to talk anecdotally or humorously about menstruation. For example, see the *The Young Ones* episode 'Interesting', which first aired 7 December 1982, for the character Rick's mistaken ideas about a tampon. Women who reached adolescence before the 1980s are unlikely to speak openly or at all about their menstrual experiences without compelling need.

Chapter 2: How not to have a baby: the history of contraception

Q: Condoms made from cloth and other substances like sheep gut were reportedly used before 1800 but not for contraceptive purposes: what were their wearers using them for?

A: Condoms were used by male customers of prostitutes in an effort to avoid contracting a sexually transmitted disease. References from contemporary sources are allusive rather than direct. The example typically cited by historians is that of James Boswell (1740–95), diarist and later biographer of Dr Samuel Johnson, who made forays into the London underworld of prostitution with or without his prophylactic 'armour' (Pottle FA editor. *Boswell's London Journal, 1762–1763*. London: 1950).

Chapter 3: 'The sperm of men is full of small children' and other early ideas about conception

Q: Why might people have been worried on theological grounds by the idea that every sperm contained a preformed human?

A: Historian Forman-Cody argues that informed commentators recoiled from the idea that multiple human lives were inevitably lost with every ejaculation (whether due to intercourse or masturbation). Christian reluctance to countenance the 'spermist' view gave rise to some stretched logic: Leeuwenhoek argued, for example, that preformed individuals (a generic act of creation) were more probable than the notion that God performed a miraculous act of creation each and every time a sperm encountered an egg.

Chapter 4: Labour: temporary pain but permanent debility?

Q: How common is it for women to suffer some degree of pelvic-organ prolapse? What are the other symptoms in addition to pain when going to the toilet, as was described in 1915?

A: According to advice issued by the NHS via the Internet, up to half of all women suffer some degree of prolapse (www.nhs.uk/conditions/Prolapse_of_the_uterus/Pages/Introduction.aspx (accessed 8 May 2013)). The symptoms can include urinary incontinence.

Chapter 5: Fashion and forceps? The medicalisation of childbirth

Q: Forceps are still unhinged but interlocking. Why?

A: It would be exceptionally difficult and probably damaging to insert ready-hinged forceps into the birth canal. Since the blades are separable, they can be inserted individually and then interlocked to secure traction. Historically, some designs of forceps included the ability to lock them in position (maintaining a fixed aperture between the blades) by means of a small nut at the point where the metal blades cross. This mechanism would prevent undue pressure from being exerted on the infant's skull by a trainee or nervous practitioner; however, most modern sets of forceps cannot be fixed in this way.

Chapter 6: How midwives became 'gamps'

Q: From your own training and practice, have you encountered present-day tensions between midwives and obstetricians? How does any conflict between the two practitioners manifest?

A: Conflicts manifest at the interpersonal and local-administrative levels. Verbal exchanges between doctors at all stages of their career (from medical students to consultants) and midwives are freighted with this history, so can be wilfully terse or obtuse in both expressive and receptive language. Each group may develop derogatory nicknames for the other, and accuse each other of minor incompetence to third parties (such as patients). Administratively, doctors tend to be senior to midwives, no matter how much their hospital structure might try to emphasise the collaborative nature of maternity healthcare, which offers the potential for doctors to assert their power officially while midwives subvert it unofficially. At the top of both professions there is a very public display of punctilious respect for one another, except when, or unless, political change encourages open expressions of surprise, concern or reproach for a perceived failure of understanding or mutual regard.

Chapter 7: The 'change': menopause and its meanings

Q: De Beauvoir wrote very frankly about women's sexuality in *The Second Sex*; to what extent did this openness translate to her autobiographical works?

A: Her memoirs skirt around the issue of her physical relationships. De Beauvoir forged a lifelong commitment with her fellow philosopher Jean Paul Sartre, but although their relationship was sexual, they did not marry and they were not exclusive. Both took lovers of both sexes, and were involved in some shared relationships and, controversially, relationships involving their underage students. Therefore, even imaginative, revealing and groundbreaking work does not necessarily tell the whole story.

Section 4: Infection, immunity and public health
Chapter 1: The 'king's evil' or 'wasting disease': tuberculosis
Q1: What was the medical significance of having a diagnostic test?

A: It was a way of identifying infected people soon after they had been infected. In addition, it allowed efficient location of sources of infection, could give an idea of the extent of the problem in a community and help to assess the effectiveness of public health measures.

Q2: Why has the prevalence of tuberculosis increased so much over the last three decades?

A: A combination of reasons has contributed to its resurgence, including drug resistance, increased global travel and HIV/acquired immune deficiency syndrome.

Chapter 2: Health and livelihood
Q1: How does each body deal with the issue of sick pay? What is the difference in the treatment of the topic between the two?

A: An assumption of patient entitlement is present for healthcare workers but not for construction workers.

Q2: What is the mid- to long-term employment/earnings outlook for a builder with a musculoskeletal disorder as opposed to a doctor who contracts hepatitis B? In either case, has the outlook changed recently?

A: The outlook for a builder who lacks private medical insurance or income-protection insurance is one of increasing impoverishment, since there is little or nothing in the way of collective trade provision for such workers suffering disablement or the consequences of curtailed employment. Furthermore state benefits are basic in Britain and may be non-existent in some countries. The medical profession is better protected by virtue of both long-standing financial supports aside from private insurance, and by recent changes to legislation. In Britain, for example, the Royal Medical Benevolent Fund exists to support practitioners in financial difficulty, and healthcare workers are no longer at risk of being barred from employment on contracting a blood-borne virus (or BBV) such as Hepatitis B. The practitioner at risk of having contracted a BBV has an obligation to be tested, and may not be able while infectious to conduct exposure-prone procedures (or EPPs), but they are not entirely prevented from working in medicine or dentistry. This sort of leeway for practitioners is a recent development. In 2000, there was little guidance available anywhere in the world about how infected practitioners should work or whether they should be permitted to work; however, in the years since the millennium, protocols for safe practice have been established (see in the British context *Health Clearance for Tuberculosis, Hepatitis B, Hepatitis C and HIV: new healthcare workers.* Department of Health; 2007).

Chapter 3: From variolation to vaccination
Q1: Wakefield's research concluded that there was a link between the MMR vaccine and autism and bowel disease. What damage did Wakefield's fraudulent research do?

A: Take-up of the vaccine decreased, which lead to MMR levels dropping to 73% of that required for herd immunity. In 2008, measles was again declared endemic in Britain, 10 years after the scare. Two children died.

Q2: Between 1885 and 1897, vaccines were developed for seven major infectious diseases. What were these?

A: Rabies, cholera, tetanus, diphtheria, anthrax, typhoid and bubonic plague.

Chapter 4: The germ theory of disease

Q: What are Koch's postulates?

A: The microorganism must be found in all organisms suffering from the disease but should not be found in healthy organisms. The microorganism must be isolated from a diseased organism and grown in pure culture. The cultured microorganism should cause disease when introduced into a healthy organism. The microorganism must be re-isolated from the inoculated diseased experimental host and identified as being identical to the original specific causative agent.

Chapter 5: Syphilis, self-pollution and stigma

Q: What has syphilis colloquially been known as in the past? What does this suggest about the potentially stigmatising nature of an obvious diagnosis?

A: Nations have tended to apportion blame for the spread of syphilis to their neighbours, opponents or enemies. Thus, in England it was known popularly as the 'French disease' while in The Netherlands it was known as the 'Spanish disease'. This suggests that stigma has historically been recognised and mobilised in the denigration of military opponents.

Chapter 6: 'Flu pandemics of the twentieth century

Q: What was it now theoretically possible to achieve?

A: Anti-viral agents and vaccines.

Chapter 8: Water as a historical force

Q: John Snow first disseminated his theory that cholera was waterborne in 1849. How did *The Lancet* and other medical journals react to his idea?

A: Medical journals were not only dismissive of Snow's theory, they also subjected it to satirical criticism. The problem for Snow was that the dominant theory of cholera transmission was anti-contagionist; this took the form of belief in air, stinks and smells or 'miasma' as the transmitting agent(s). When Snow offered his alternative theory, medical authorities assumed he must be in league with organisations who stood to gain from any reduction of the focus on smell (such as industries like tanning that produced powerful stenches in their vicinity). Snow's problem was that microscopy could not deliver proof in the 1850s of waterborne bacteria. Snow died in 1858, 8 years before his theory became more widely accepted and over 20 years before the identification of the bacillus responsible (in the 1880s).

Section 5: The challenges of life: childhood, disability, ageing and mental illness

Chapter 2: Two steps forward, one step back: disability

Q1: What benefits are available to those with disability in England and Wales?

A: At the time of writing, the Disability Living Allowance had just been changed to the Personal Independence Payment. The Disability Living Allowance was made up of two components, mobility and care, and the maximum someone could qualify for was £131.50 per week.

Q2: What was the aim of Aktion T4 in 1939?

A: Aktion T4 was referred to as the 'euthanasia programme' after the Second World War. It aimed to exterminate mentally and physically disabled people and officially ran from 1939 to 1941, although it continued to 1945. In 1941, Clemens von Galen (1878–1946), a Catholic priest, delivered a series of excoriating sermons in Münster Cathedral attacking the Nazi programme on euthanasia, forced sterilisation and concentration camps. His sermons were copied and sent to German soldiers on the Western and Eastern Fronts. As a result, although Aktion T4 continued, it did so with greater secrecy. By 1945, it is estimated that at least 200000 people had been killed by starvation, in the gas chambers or by experimental medication. Hitler's personal physician led the programme.

Q3: What is the Snellen test?

A: The Snellen test measures visual acuity by asking patients to read progressively smaller letters on a chart from a certain distance. Created by Hermann Snellen in 1862, the chart consists of 11 lines of letters beginning at the top with one large letter followed by lines with increasing numbers of letters, with the letters in each line smaller than in the line before. The last line that the individual can read accurately determines acuity for that eye.

Chapter 3: Broken bones and failing joints

Q: Would you agree with these statements?

A: Gout is a condition that affects post-pubertal males more than females. When women acquire it, they tend to be on average 60 years old, that is 10 years older than men who develop it. Acute episodes are more common in the spring. Inflammation, which is acutely painful, subsides within a few days.

Chapter 4: Ageing and the good death

Q1: What happened to older people who were poor before the twentieth century?

A: Following the Poor Law of 1601, each parish was required to levy funds to care for the destitute who were considered 'deserving', which included older people. In 1834, relief was withdrawn from all those deemed capable of being engaged in productive work; those who were destitute were sent to frugal and punitive establishments, the workhouses. In theory, older people were meant to reside in separate accommodation but provision was variable, so they also ended up in the dreaded workhouses. By 1900, their plight was so dire that Poor Law unions were obliged to provide comfortable and separate accommodation for older people where husbands and wives could lie together.

Q2: What changes have since occurred that may have improved the care of older people and the dying?

A: Changes include: the development of the 'geriatrics' speciality, after the term was introduced by Ignatz Nascher (1863–1945) in the early twentieth century, who recognised the need for a specialism in the diseases of old age; increasing expertise in palliative care; increasing interest in the psychological needs of the dying and the process of bereavement; demographic changes and the rise of the 'grey' lobby; and a backlash against impersonalised, non-compassionate medicalisation of death.

Chapter 5: What price immortality?

Q1: Should O'Byrne's wishes finally be heeded and his remains buried, or should his bones be retained as a focus of display and study?

A: There is no easy answer to this, particularly given that O'Byrne has not been a focus of Irish anti-English dissatisfaction (so, at the time of writing, there is no widespread agitation for the bones to be buried) and that the skeleton currently holds pride of place at the heart of the Hunterian Museum. The argument is not simply a pragmatic one, however; there is a trend for people in the present to apologise for events in the past, undertaken in a different moral climate. Why else would the city of Liverpool have 'apologised' in 1999 for the city's role in the Atlantic slave trade? You decide.

Q2: Do you think any restitution is owed to the Lacks family or should the individual's story be subordinate to the achievements of successful tissue culture and its therapeutic applications? Does your reaction to the story change when you learn that Lacks was African-American?

A: In terms of natural justice, the surviving children of Henrietta Lacks (or their direct descendants) should clearly be offered some form of settlement for the use of Henrietta's cells; however, the family has not tried to sue anyone for their use of the cells, and their legal position would not be strong if they tried. In any event, they do not wish to see research using HeLa cells to end but they hope, in the words of one of Henrietta's sons, that 'Hopkins and some of the other folks who benefited off her cells will do something to honor her and make right with the family.' For the context of this quote and further guidance on debates about tissue retention in the USA until 2009, see the afterword in Rebecca Skloot's book about Lacks, listed in the 'Further reading' section of this chapter.

Race was and is a potent social signifier in the USA. Lacks' status as the wife and daughter of poor, black tobacco farmers who died before the start of the civil rights movement adds yet another layer of disadvantage and exploitation to her story.

Q3: In your opinion, who or what was most responsible for the public outcry: individual medical practitioners, hospital administrators, the tabloid press, procedural inertia in the NHS or some other factor?

A: Clearly, in matters of opinion, there can be no definitive answer. However, it is notable that the newspaper and television media have been quick to blame (and to continue to blame) practitioners and hospital cultures, while practitioners themselves tend to allude defensively to misunderstandings between the doctors involved, historical anatomy practice (which routinely involved harvesting organ and tissue samples) and patient perceptions. See, in particular, the websites of the BBC, *The Guardian*, *Daily Mail* and other British newspapers as well as the hospital's own site for varying responses to the story (for example www.guardian. co.uk and www.dailymail.co.uk).

Chapter 7: Mind and brain

Q: Can you think of some examples?

A: Concepts with widespread cultural currency include defence mechanisms such as displacement and repression; the unconscious; the id, ego and superego; unresolved conflicts; and the inferiority complex.

Section 6: Practising medicine: diagnostic methods

Chapter 1: Early Greek and Roman contributions

Q: Are there any examples in current biomedical knowledge of the number four being significant?

A: The genetic code consists of four nucleic bases, adenine, guanine, cytosine and thymine. Each is constituted from a mixture of four elements: carbon, oxygen, hydrogen and nitrogen.

Chapter 2: '[T]he most liquid evacuations imaginable': excreta as a diagnostic aid

Q1: How are anal fistulae managed today?

A: A simple fistula is treated by a surgical procedure called a 'fistulotomy'. A 'seton' may be used, which is a surgical thread left in the opened fistula tract to keep the tract open and improve drainage. Complex fistulae are more difficult to treat successfully because of the risk of incontinence. The usual operation is advancement flap repair with adequate tract drainage. New sphincter-preserving techniques include using a bio-prosthetic plug to block the internal opening of the fistula.

Q2: What illnesses are characterised by this symptom?

A: One of the most serious illnesses that features watery diarrhoea is cholera (*see* Section 4, Chapter 8, 'Water as a historical force').

Chapter 3: The rise of modern medicine: the evolution of modern physical diagnosis

Q: Who developed these instruments and what reception did they have?

A: Hermann von Helmholtz (1821–94) invented the ophthalmoscope. Carl Wunderlich (1815–77) invented the thermometer, which measured changes of temperature on a scale – the thermoscope had been used since the sixteenth century but only indicated a change in temperature. Use of the reflex hammer was popularised by Wilhelm Erb (1840–1921).

Like the technique of percussion, these new instruments were often initially viewed with scepticism, so it was some time before they were widely adopted.

Chapter 4: The beat, beat, beat of the drum: the discovery of circulation and the tools to measure it

Q: How did measuring blood pressure improve medical practice? What measurement was yet to be routinely recorded and who devised the technique for doing so?

A: Cushing used blood pressure measurements during surgical operations to monitor patients' physical status. Frederick Mahomed (c. 1849–84), a physician at Guy's Hospital, London, measured his scarlet fever patients' blood pressure and showed that a sudden increase in blood pressure was a symptom of impending acute nephritis. He pioneered the habit of taking regular blood pressure recordings to ascertain a patient's progress.

Chapter 5: From toy to tool: the microscope

Q: Who were these scientists and what did they demonstrate?

A: Rudolf Virchow (1821–1902) founded the discipline of cellular pathology and encouraged his medical students 'to think microscopically' (Schultz M. Robert

Virchow. *Emeg. Infect. Dis.* 2008. **14**(9) 1480–81.) Together with others, he was a firm exponent of 'cell theory', which states that cells are the basic units of life and their division leads to new cells. He rejected the concept of 'spontaneous generation', which held that living organisms could emerge from non-living matter. Ferdinand Cohn (1828–98) made a systematic classification of bacteria and popularised the use of the microscope in microbiology. His work also helped to disprove spontaneous generation. Louis Pasteur (1822–95) demonstrated that microorganisms are present in the air and are responsible for disease. Robert Koch (1843–1910), with the aid of new staining methods, distinguished microbes and identified a number of pathogens by the end of the nineteenth century (*see* Section 4, Chapter 4, 'The germ theory of disease').

Section 7: Practising medicine: interventions and cures

Chapter 1: The appeal of the miracle cure

Q: How was mercury administered to patients – orally, anally or topically?

A: Mercury was sold in pill form for oral use, as an ointment and sometimes as a preparation for bathing in. These forms of treatment had a noticeable effect on the skin lesions caused by syphilis but did little to address the underlying infection. Further, prolonged exposure was likely to cause mercury poisoning.

Chapter 2: Medical misdirection

Q1: What developments occurred to discredit bloodletting as a standard treatment?

A: Aside from the general decline of humoral theory that underpinned the act of letting blood, at least three factors led to its being discredited.

1. Dr Pierre Louis studied patients diagnosed with pneumonia, comparing their survival rates on the basis of when they had been subjected to bloodletting. He concluded that survival rate was much lower if the patient had undergone bloodletting in the early phase of illness [first 3 days] when the patient was very ill, compared to a later phase [7–9 days] when the patient was probably improving.

2. By the end of the nineteenth century, there was a better understanding of physiology and microbiology, together with an acceptance of the germ theory of disease.

3. The clinical observation that bloodletting was entirely inappropriate for patients with a weakened physical status.

Q2: We may be amused at some of these treatments, but there has been renewed interest in the therapeutic uses of electricity in the twentieth and twenty-first centuries. For what conditions has it been revived?

A: Deep brain, occipital and transcranial magnetic stimulation for migraine and transcranial magnetic stimulation for severe depression, as an alternative to electroconvulsive therapy.

Chapter 3: The rise of pharmacology: a story of prepared minds, money and serendipity

Q1: Boyle is often considered the father of chemistry. What is he remembered for?

A: Boyle introduced an approach to scientific inquiry that we would recognise as modern because he employed observation, experiment and rational thought. With

Robert Hooke (1635–1703), he built an air pump to produce a vacuum and demonstrated that air was essential to life. Boyle also demonstrated that there is an inverse relationship between the volume of a gas and its pressure (Boyle's law) and showed that a compound material can have different properties to its constituents.

Q2: What other infections did sulphonamides help to cure?

A: Principally erysipelas, scarlet fever and puerperal fever; use of sulphonamides for the latter, which is due to streptococcal infection, saw the mortality rate fall from 2.5 per 1000 births in 1937 to 0.5 per 1000 births in 1940.

Q3: What was serendipitous about the discovery of insulin?

A: In 1889, Oskar Minkowski (1858–1931) hypothesised that something in the pancreas must regulate metabolism and thereby prevent diabetes mellitus. Thirty years later, Canadian surgeon Frederick Banting (1891–1941) experimented on dogs. After ligating the pancreatic ducts, he removed the pancreas once the acini had died. When the animals became glycosuric, he administered extracts of degenerated pancreas. By this time, the advances that had taken place in blood glucose estimation enabled him to monitor the dogs' diabetic condition. On giving the extract, he found that the dogs' blood glucose reduced. He was able to undertake these experiments because John JR Macleod (1876–1935), a professor of physiology and an expert in carbohydrate metabolism, allowed him to use a small part of his laboratory and supplied him a student to help, Charles Best (1899–1978). The addition of a third team member, James Collip (1892–1965), a biochemist, helped tighten up the research and enabled the development of a method for purifying the extract without which the enterprise would probably have failed. Ironically, Macleod initially thought that Banting's work would not succeed and that it would be helpful to have this negative finding. Later collaboration with the Eli Lilly company helped to overcome the difficulty of manufacturing large quantities of insulin for routine use in medicine.

Q4: What were the consequences to the pharmaceutical industry of this tragedy?

A: Safety regulations became stricter with regard to the testing of new drugs. From 1969, in Britain it became mandatory to test toxicity on animals and for the drug to undergo several stages of clinical trials on humans before it could be released to the public. By 1978 the 'development time' for a new drug had increased by 10 years. By the 1990s, costs had escalated 30-fold. The rate of innovation over those 30 years declined. This was partly but not wholly attributable to regulatory changes. In 1964, 3 years after thalidomide was withdrawn in Britain, the World Medical Association's Declaration of Helsinki put greater ethical strictures on clinical research.

Chapter 4: From party games to pain control: the early story of anaesthesia

Q: What do think were the reasonable medical concerns about the new anaesthetics?

A: Chloroform proved to result in a high mortality rate. The first death was that of 15-year-old Hannah Greener in 1848. Ether was 10 times safer but caused several side effects such as coughing, nausea and vomiting, and excessive salivation. It was also highly flammable, which was a real concern in an age when candles were used for illumination. Nitrous oxide was not strong enough for use as a general anaesthetic.

Chapter 5: Transplantation

Q1: Why would it be difficult to continue operating with such a high failure rate in contemporary medical practice?

A: Audit of practice is now embedded in the NHS. 'Audit' involves the measuring of practice against agreed treatment standards and implementing change to ensure all patients receive care to the same standard. The royal colleges in Britain started carrying out systematic audits on clinical practice in the 1970s. Medical audit was formally introduced in 1989 in the Department of Health's paper *Working for Patients*, which advocated systematic peer review of medical care and required that audit should be part of routine clinical practice of all doctors. It soon became apparent that for audit to be effective, it had to be embraced by all the health disciplines.

Q2: What other advances helped to improve the survival rate among transplant patients?

A: Another immunosuppressant, cyclosporine, was discovered, which was more effective than azathioprine and reduced the amount of steroids needed.

Chapter 6: Cutting for stone: the hazards of surgery

Q1: Bladder stones are a less common complaint in the twentieth century. Why?

A: Simply, because of an improved and more variable diet.

Q2: How did antiseptic surgery come about?

A: A Hungarian obstetrician, Ignaz Semmelweis (1818–65), noticed that the mortality rate due to puerperal fever, which was very common at the time, was much worse in one of two lying-in wards for women at the Vienna General Hospital where he was working. Initially, he could find no difference between the wards but eventually realised that one was used for teaching midwives and the other for medical students. Then, when a friend died after an accidental injury from a scalpel during a post-mortem, he concluded that the medical students who regularly attended post-mortems must be carrying 'cadaverous particles' on their hands, which caused the puerperal fever. Therefore, from 1847, he insisted that they and all others attending the women wash their hands first with chlorinated lime. The mortality rate reduced to just 1%. He did not publish his findings until 1858 (*The Aetiology of Childbed Fever*) although former students disseminated his ideas. His discovery was mainly dismissed partly because his paper was misunderstood and partly because of his failure to provide a satisfactory explanation as to why his methods worked. The germ theory of disease had not yet been discovered (*see* Section 4, Chapter 4, 'The germ theory of disease') and it is said that his colleagues took exception to being asked to wash their hands since this implied that, although they were 'gentlemen', they were somehow unclean. When Pasteur published his work demonstrating that microorganisms spread infection, it occurred to a British surgeon, Joseph Lister (1827–1912), that wound infections might be caused by them. He experimented with various dilutions of carbolic acid swabbed on wound sites to eliminate any microorganisms and presented his findings to the British Medical Association in 1867, which were well received. By the 1880s, Lister, along with most surgeons, favoured an aseptic technique to produce a sterile surgical environment.

Section 8: Healers and health carers

Chapter 1: From spicer to pharmacist

Q: A further tragic scandal occurred in the early 1960s. What was this and what was the legislative response?

A: The scandal involved the drug thalidomide, which led to thousands of mothers giving birth to deformed babies in Western Europe (*see* Section 7, Chapter 3, 'The rise of pharmacology: a story of prepared minds, money and serendipity'). The drug was not available in the USA, but the public was alarmed and supported stronger drug regulation, which soon instigated legislation for the review of all drugs already being prescribed for their safety and efficacy.

Chapter 2: Diminishing Nightingale: an alternative history of nursing

Q: By how much was the mortality rate at Scutari Hospital, Istanbul, reduced in the 6 months after the arrival of Nightingale and her group of 38 nurses?

A: This is a trick question; the mortality rate in Scutari rose in the first 6 months of Nightingale's appointment but fell rather sharply thereafter, from over 30% to below 10%.

Chapter 3: The origins of physiotherapy

Q: Why is polio not a major health concern today in the Western world?

A: During another epidemic in the 1950s, Dr Jonas Salk (1914–95) reported a series of successful tests using a killed vaccine. Although his vaccine was safe, it was less effective than a live attenuated virus. By 1964, following significant trials, three types of effective and safe vaccine were available that were successfully widely disseminated. One continuing difficulty today, however, is that of maintaining high immunity levels in developing, politically unstable, countries.

Chapter 4: The shifting sands of health management

Q1: What has been the consequence of the establishment of the NHS in the UK?

A: The provision of reasonable health services to the whole population, irrespective of class or income *and* the involvement of the government in a wide range of areas previously considered the responsibility of private citizens. However, some have seen the establishment of the NHS as the creation of a behemoth that has required an increasing share of the country's resources to fund.

Q2: What has been the consequence of central government increasingly seeking to micro-manage the NHS?

A: A significant improvement in the quality of service provision and rational allocation of resources, alongside an explosion of focus on performance targets and an army of managers to deliver and analyse them. Arguably, this has entailed an undermining of the ethos of public service, as managers, whose jobs depend on attainment of targets, have learned to 'manage' results to demonstrate such attainment.

Index

Index

Index

Index

medical history
  ownership of 5–6
  value of 3–5
medical humanities 1–2, 5
medical insurance schemes 24
medical knowledge 4, 22, 143–4, 147, 172
medical research
  challenging orthodoxy 108, 158
  ethics in 96, 129
medical tourism 39
medical witnesses 23
medicine, dialogue with history 1–2
menopause 75–6, 124, 212
menstrual blood 51, 61, 75
menstruation
  and anaemia 51
  euphemisms for 61–2
mental illness
  physical treatments for 136–7
  social attitudes to 130–4
  therapy for 131–2
  and warfare 30
mercury
  administration of 218
  and syphilis 95, 97, 165
mescal 46
mesmerism 167, 169, 179
miasma 80, 214
microscopes
  and blood circulation 156
  development of 159–61
  and germ theory of disease 92–3
  and pathological changes 152
midwives 23, 70–1, 73–4, 192, 212, 220
migraine 168, 218
mind, location and nature of 135–6, 138
mind-altering drugs 44, 46–7
mining, health and safety in 18–20
Minkowski, Oskar 219
miracle cures 138, 165–6, 218
MMR vaccine 89, 213
monastic orders 191, 202
Montagu, Mary 87–8
Morgagni, Giovanni Battista 152
morphine 47, 126, 171, 173
mortality rates, publication of 12
Morton, William TG 178
motor vehicles 15–16, 208
motorcycles 208
Munk, William 125
Murray, Joseph 183–4
Myers, Charles 209

National Insurance 84
Nazi Germany
  and eugenics 42, 133
  euthanasia in 115, 215
  medical experiments in 174–5
  smoking in 209
needle phobia 14
Newton, Isaac 173
NHS (National Health Service)
  audit of practice in 220
  dental care on 38–9
  establishment of 202–3, 221
  history of 6
  liability of 24
  management of 203–5
  and mental illness 130, 137
NICE (National Institute for Health and Care
  Excellence) 5
Nidana 87
Nigeria 53
Nightingale, Florence 79, 196–8, 221
Nightingale Fund 197
Nihell, Elizabeth 71
nitrous oxide 82, 177–8, 219
Noel, Walter Clement 54
noses, remodelling 186
NSPCC (National Society for the Prevention
  of Cruelty to Children) 111–12
nursing
  history of 196–8
  profession of 203

obstetricians 72–3, 212
O'Byrne, Charles 128, 216
ogbanje 53–4
old age
  and disability 117
  and resuscitation 27
  use of term 123–4
ophthalmoscope 153, 217
opiates
  as pain control 177
  in patent medicines 165
  sale of 45
opium 44–6, 120, 125, 132, 177
organs
  diseased 152
  for donation 185
  harvesting of 129, 216
orthodoxy, contradicting 108
orthopaedics 119, 199–200
Orwell, George 79

Index

CPD with Radcliffe

You can now use a selection of our books to achieve CPD (Continuing Professional Development) points through directed reading.

We provide a free online form and downloadable certificate for your appraisal portfolio. Look for the CPD logo and register with us at: www.radcliffehealth.com/cpd

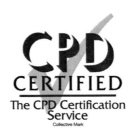